The Stretch

Simple Exercises to Improve Flexibility, Increase Mobility and Relieve Tension

By Dale L. Roberts

©2015

The Stretch Workout Plan: Simple Exercises to Improve Flexibility, Increase Mobility & Relieve Tension

DISCLAIMER

This book proposes a program of exercise recommendations. However, all readers must consult a qualified medical professional before starting this or any other health & fitness program. As with any exercise program, if you experience any discomfort, pain or duress of any sort, stop immediately and consult your physician. This book is intended for an audience that is free of any health condition, physical limitation or injury. The creators, producers, participants, advertisers and distributors of this program disclaim any liabilities or losses in connection with the exercises or advice herein. Any equipment or workout area that is used should be thoroughly inspected ahead of use as free of danger, flaw or compromise. The user assumes all responsibility when performing any movements contained in this book and waives the equipment manufacturer, makers, and distributors of the equipment of all liabilities.

Table of Contents

Introduction

With internet headlines like *The Dangers of Stretching*[1], *The Truth Behind 7 Muscle Myths: Stretching Prevents Injuries*[2] and *Center for Disease Control: Stretching Causes Muscle Injuries*[3], the importance of stretching is lost on more people than ever. Though these disruptive headlines command your attention, the content reveals a common theme - stretching is good for you. Yet, stretching comes with precautions to maximize benefits and to decrease risks.

In *The Stretch Workout Plan*, I reveal the truth behind stretching and why most everyone benefits from it. Stretching isn't simply great for relieving muscle tension and soreness but also improves blood flow, decreases stress, and develops better posture[4]. And, your quality of life is affected by two crucial elements, flexibility and mobility.

This book provides a better understanding of proper stretching by considering two key factors - timing and type. Timing is in knowing when and how long to stretch for the most safety and effectiveness. Equally important is the type of stretch to affect a particular area of the body.

I include plenty of stretches with a variety of techniques to keep you excited and eager to try out a new exercise every day. Each stretch exercise comes with brief instructions on how to perform the movement and what part of the body it affects. Every stretch and position come with different techniques so you have more than one way to do the exercise.

More important than learning how simple stretching is, you must apply the knowledge afterward. Take a little time every day to practice a new stretch, and when you perfect it, move on to the next one. Keep adding one stretch exercise to your daily routine and you will reap the rewards. In due time, you will discover *The Stretch Workout Plan* is an excellent way to enhance your quality of life through simple, yet effective, exercises done most anywhere at any time. Now let's get loosened up!

"Knowledge is of no value unless you put it into practice."
-Anton Chekhov, Russian physician & author

Simplicity in Stretching

Starting or changing a fitness routine is challenging enough, so I promise stretching won't be complicated. You won't become a contortionist or advanced yogi by following my instructions. What you will get from this book is an understanding of why and how you should stretch. First, you should know a few key terms appearing throughout the book. These words give you a better grasp of all the exercises and how they benefit you.

Flexibility

Flexibility is the ability of your muscle or your body part to relax and allow stretch and stress forces[5]. Certain factors influence your flexibility, such as age, gender or physical activity. The amount of flexibility will determine the range of motion or the full movement potential of a joint[6].

The range of motion, or the degree of movement, at a joint is affected by your muscles, tendons, ligaments, and bones. Every joint has a unique function and should only move through specific movement sequences. Some joints are meant to bend through a minimum range of motion to keep the muscles, tendons and ligaments active, and, therefore, preventing atrophy or excess tension. Through consistent stretching, you can maintain an ideal range of motion. When you learn fundamental stretch exercises, you can train your body to move and feel better.

According to the U.S. National Library of Medicine, flexibility diminishes with age.[7] Natural degenerative changes occur, including joints becoming stiffer and less pliable. Fluid in the joints decrease and cartilage gets worn away. Normal aging creates change in the muscle and the nervous system, causing the muscle to have less toning and ability to contract. The muscle becomes more rigid and less toned, even with regular exercise. With the proper medical consultation, senior citizens can develop a daily stretch routine for maintaining the quality of life based on their specific health conditions.

Another interesting fact is females are more flexible than males. Individual research studies performed by *The Canadian Journal of Applied Sport Sciences* (Bell/Hoshizaki, 1981, Dec. 6) and *Ergonomics* (Doriot/Wang, 2006, Feb. 22) separately found that women have a significantly greater range of motion than men.[89] The study found the female body has minor differences in joint structure and connective tissue (i.e. muscle, tendons, and ligaments) than the male body[10], permitting the increased degree of movement.

Physical activity plays another important part of flexibility. According to a study by the National Center for Biotechnology, more physically active people have better flexibility than non-active individuals.[11] A sedentary lifestyle, or lots of sitting and inactivity, contributes to stiff joints and a shorter range of motion.[12] Of course, not all activity improves overall flexibility. In fact, certain repetitive movements lead to muscular imbalances creating discomfort, pain or even injury. Properly stretching overworked muscles helps restore muscular balance and may decrease the risk of injury.[13]

Mobility

Mobility is the ability to move with ease and without restriction[14]. Your overall flexibility determines the extent of your mobility or the degree of your total movements. For instance, the mobility of a person who walks upright compared to someone who walks slouched-over indicates a difference in flexibility limitations.

Through stretching, you can address inflexible areas and gain better mobility. Correct any muscular imbalances through flexibility training and you can increase your overall mobility. Any significant mobility impairments can affect quality of life.[15]

The Danger of Muscle Tension

Soreness and tightness usually accompany most workouts, repetitive activities and lack of movement. Overuse and underuse can wreak havoc on the body and while balance can be difficult, it is still possible.

Most people feel a sense of accomplishment when they are sore or have muscle tension after a great workout. The soreness validates a job well done, but, in actuality, this indicates small tears in the muscle fiber. Adequate hydration, good nutrition, and proper stretching can help repair and rebuild torn muscle fibers. If this soreness isn't addressed, the body recognizes it as a threat and begins to compensate for this issue. Your body will overcompensate in another area and decrease mobility until a correction in the perceived injury.

Repetitive activities in the workplace can play a huge part in mobility limitations. For instance, assembly line jobs that require repeated movement can cause cramping and tension in the overused muscles. Most assembly line jobs include a method of grabbing, picking or pulling that overuse the forearm, wrist, and biceps. This repetition shortens the muscles and eventually creates discomfort, spasms or injury. If this isn't addressed early, then it may lead to injuries, such as muscle tears, strains or sprains.[16]

Lastly, a sedentary lifestyle, or being inactive, is the worst for your mobility. By limiting your activity, you hinder your mobility and become a lot more inflexible. Lack of movement creates atrophy or a wasting away of muscle.

The solution to muscle tension is consistent stretching.

Stretching

Stretching is an exercise in pulling a body part away from its anatomically neutral position[17] or your natural, relaxed position. Through proper stretching with the right amount of force and consistent efforts, benefits include:

1. returning muscle to its resting state after exercise[18]
2. maintain joint range of motion[19]
3. provide temporary relief from exercise-induced soreness[20]
4. decrease potential of injury[21]
5. improve blood circulation with some stretches[22]
6. burn more calories than at rest[23]
7. improve posture[24]

Knowing the 3 types of stretching and when to do them is important for you to reap the rewards. Otherwise, you increase the likelihood of injury when doing the wrong kinds of stretches at the wrong time[25].

Types & Timing of Stretching

Static, dynamic and ballistic stretching are the three types of stretching. This chapter primarily covers static stretching—the simplest form of flexibility training. I briefly discuss dynamic stretching and how it's more than holding or rapidly dipping in and out of a position. Then, I explain the dated concept and dangers of ballistic stretching.

Additionally, I recommend a few inexpensive fitness tools to enhance your flexibility training. Some stretch tools are, as simple as, a chair or wall. Other tools have a small cost, like straps or foam rollers.

As with any type of fitness activity, stretching comes with a few precautions for safety and effectiveness. The articles I listed in the introduction are correct in the implications of danger. People with special needs, conditions and injuries need to consult their doctor before beginning these stretch exercises. Read all the way through the book before starting any of this routine to see if stretching is appropriate for you.

Static Stretching

The type of stretch primarily covered in this book is static meaning to hold in place[26]. In static stretching, you move into a position and hold. Even though static stretching is the most commonly used type of flexibility training, it is also the most misunderstood and misused form of exercise. Research has shown a pre-workout static stretch routine does not improve exercise performance, increase blood flow or decrease the likelihood of injury[27][28]. So, static stretching is not an adequate warm-up for the body. The best time for static stretching is after a workout or as a standalone routine.

A few static stretch methods include:

1) Static passive - An outside force or object is used to assist with applying the stretch. This type of stretch is great for all fitness levels.
Timing: Hold position for 20-30 seconds. After the first 7 seconds, relax the targeted area and sink deeper into the stretch. It's okay if you can't stretch further—practice makes perfect.
Example: When you bend and touch your toes, you are doing so without the effort of activating your muscles to get into position.

Also, using a strap to pull your body into a position is a static passive stretch.

2) Static active - The strength of one muscle group is used to hold the stretched muscle in place. This type of stretch is for experienced exercisers since it requires more balance, body position awareness and control.

Timing: Hold position for 5-10 seconds at a time.

Example: From a standing position you extend one leg out in front you and hold it. This is a static active stretch. It requires the muscle on the front of your leg to stretch the muscle on the back of your leg.

3) Isometric - This is also known as a static contraction of a muscle. An isometric stretch is when you get into a stretch position, then contract the stretched muscle. This stretch should be used with caution and with supervision if you aren't experienced. You may injure your tendons, ligaments or joints if you contract the stretched muscle too much. Isometric stretching is not recommended for anyone under 18 years old. Once again, this type of stretch is for more experienced exercisers.

Timing: Get into position, and then contract the affected area for 10-15 seconds. Repeat this movement 2-5 times for the best results.

Example: Any exercise can be used as an example when you just hold position and your muscles contract to keep still.

4) Proprioceptive neuromuscular facilitation (PNF) - Considered the best stretch for improving joint range of motion, the PNF stretch is a blend of static passive and isometric stretching. PNF stretching requires a trained professional to assist the movement safely. The pro moves a person's body part to a point of mild discomfort. This passive stretch is held for 10 seconds. On instruction, the person pushes against the professional's hand. The person should apply just enough force so that the body part remains static. The hold lasts for 6 seconds. The athlete then relaxes as the professional completes a second passive stretch held for 30 seconds. The body part should move further than before. Another way is for the professional to have the active muscle complete its full range of motion in a contracted state, then relax as the part is moved back into position.

Timing & Example: For the sake of safety, please have your doctor refer you to the best professional for your particular needs.

Dynamic Stretching

Dynamic stretching is movement-specific exercises that warm up the muscles and prepare the body for specific activities.[29] This type of stretch uses a slow, controlled movement using multiple muscle groups within their range of motion. Dynamic stretches help lubricate joints and increase muscle temperature and is the one exception to stretching as a pre-workout routine[30].

Since the vast number of dynamic stretches would take up volumes of books, I only touch on this topic. Essentially, most traditional bodyweight exercises are dynamic flexibility exercises when you go through the full range of motion at a slower pace than usual. Excellent examples of dynamic stretching are in *Component 1: Warm-Up* of *The 90-Day Home Workout Program*.

Join a fitness club, gym or private studio that hosts classes for Yoga, Tai Chi or Qigong (pronounced chi-gong). These group classes have dynamic and static stretch exercises for developing flexibility and mobility. An experienced instructor provides verbal and visual cues, as well as, encouragement while making adjustments according to your fitness level.

You may notice soreness or muscle fatigue after your workout sessions. There are two types of muscle soreness:

1. Post-workout muscle soreness that quickly fades after a session
2. Delayed onset muscle soreness (DOMS) is the soreness felt 24-48 hours after a workout. This condition is believed to be caused by microscopic tears in the connective tissue in the muscle following intense exercise sessions[31].

Stretching is one of many ways to alleviate the tension from DOMS. However, this is only a temporary fix and has not been proven to aid or speed up recovery[32]. At the very least, you may relieve tension and maintain your joint range of motion right after a workout.

Injury prevention is currently thought to be a benefit in stretching, but no scientific evidence confirms this theory.[33] Some research studies have shown no decrease in exercise injury prevention and some institutions have even hypothesized that pre-workout static stretching may actually increase your likelihood of injury, or at a minimum, diminish exercise performance.[34][35]

However, flexibility training is exercise, so you burn more calories stretching than you do at rest. If you find you need a day off from intense exercising or a great way to ease yourself into working out, then stretching is an excellent alternative as a standalone routine.

Stretching can sometimes counteract any stiffness you have from chronic and repetitive positions or movements. For instance, office workers spend their day seated at a desk, so they would benefit from regular stretching to extend the shortened muscles in the front of the body. Their focus would be on the front hips, shoulders, chest and neck since these areas tend to be in a collapsed and rested state throughout the work day[36].

Ballistic Stretching

Absolutely under no circumstances should you use ballistic stretching. This form of stretching uses the same positioning of static stretching but employs a rapid bouncing in and out of the position. Ballistic stretching can damage muscles, tendons and ligaments due to the protective nature of the stretch reflex.

Also, called the myotatic reflex, this reaction is an automatic muscle contraction to a sudden change in muscle length. The more sudden the change, the more the stretch reflex engages to protect the muscle. To avoid triggering the stretch reflex, you always should ease in and out of all stretches. The slower you move, the less apt the stretch reflex activates.

In ballistic stretching, the stretch reflex nerves do not have time to properly disengage due to the rapid movement. Therefore, the muscles you want to stretch don't adequately relax and are more susceptible to tears, sprains, strains and other more severe injuries.[37] Be cautious and avoid ballistic stretching altogether.

Stretch Strap

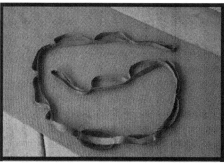

A strap is an excellent tool used to enhance static stretching. A flexibility routine should not solely rely on this device, but you can add the strap intermittently for variety in your routine. As with all stretching, apply only enough pressure on the muscle to feel some tension. The stretch should be slightly uncomfortable at worst yet never painful.

The strap can be picked up at any number of in-store or online retailers for $5 to $15, depending on the distributor. I prefer one with various loops. If you don't have the money, then you can substitute the stretch strap with a towel. Some stretches with the strap are not as easy to do if you use a towel.

The stretch strap is not a necessity and you can still adequately perform the stretch routine without this tool. A word of warning: Avoid using this tool to apply too much tension. More pressure does not mean greater improvements in flexibility. Use this tool with care and pay close attention to your body when using it.

Foam Rolling

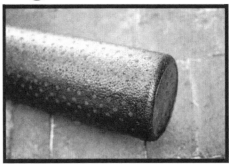

A foam roller complements your stretch routine or any workout. This device is used for self-myofascial release (SMR) or a form of self-massage. Myo- means muscle and -fascia refers to the connective tissue that wraps and bundles muscle together. A myofascial adhesion, or scar tissue, is caused by stress, training, overuse, under-use, movement imbalances or injuries[38]. This type of scar tissue can be identified as knots in your muscle that cause discomfort. The scar tissue can restrict the movement of myofascia and the overall mobility of the person[39].

Foam rolling is like massaging yourself. With some of your body weight on the foam roller, you roll over the knotted muscle. In essence, you break up trigger points and soothe tight fascia while increasing blood flow and circulation to the area[40].

How to Foam Roll

Ease yourself into these foam rolling exercises, because SMR is physically demanding. Depending on the size of a knot and the tightness of the muscle, SMR can be uncomfortable or mildly painful at worst. If you experience any pain, ease up and lift your weight off the area. Stop immediately if you experience any sharp pain and consult your family doctor.

Get into position and slowly ease your weight onto the foam roller. Gently roll away from your feet, and then toward your head. As you move, take note of the toughest area or the knots in the muscle. When you have found the knot, hold your position on top of the knot for 20-30 seconds. You may have some discomfort, but if it escalates to pain, lift some pressure from the area. Too much pressure will not allow the area to relax. Once the area has relaxed, roll above, below, and then through the knot 5-10 times each.

There are different types of foam rollers varying in density. Choose a softer low-density foam roller until you comfortably perform the exercises in this book. Switch to a thicker density foam roller when you feel fewer benefits from the low-density foam roller. Many companies manufacture at least three varieties in soft, medium and hard density foam rollers. A thicker density does not indicate physical superiority nor does it break any world records. If you find a foam roller density works for you, then keep using it.

Some people need a hard foam roller on some areas, but a lower density foam roller on other more delicate areas. For instance, I use a thick density foam roller on my back but have to use a softer density on my tight outer thighs. A thicker density foam roller doesn't work on an excessively tight area since the muscle won't relax.

You may feel an immediate difference after your first use. And, with consistent use of the foam roller, you may help relieve problematic areas and eliminate chronic adhesions. Prioritize your time on problem areas and then focus on other areas you plan to work during your exercise routine or sporting activity.

Evidence has shown that foam rolling is best used after any exercise routine or activity for its benefits. In March 2001, the National Strength and Conditioning Association conducted three studies on the effects of foam rolling on performance, recovery, range of motion and blood flow. The first test was on the impact of foam rolling on performance and recovery. Surprisingly, the study showed foam rolling had no impact on performance when done before an exercise. However, the test proved fatigue and recovery were improved by using a foam roller after exercise.[41]

The second test showed foam rolling improved joint range of motion while no adverse effects occurred in muscle performance.[42] A huge reason why I include foam rolling as a component in flexibility training is because this study indicated that foam rolling improves flexibility and mobility.

The last study showed that foam rolling improved blood circulation throughout the body. [43] Even though prior research showed no improvement in performance using SMR before a workout, this study proved that foam rolling could still prepare and warm up the body.

I recommend using foam rolling before a stretch session for the body to fully warm up and to loosen up any knots that may inhibit a deeper stretch. However, there are going to be some health conditions and populations that should not use foam rolling.

Foam Rolling Warning

Foam rolling should never be used if you have osteoarthritis, osteoporosis, blood pressure issues or are on any blood thinner medications.[44] Due to the positioning requirements, avoid foam rolling if you have any back problems or prior injuries. If you have difficulty supporting your bodyweight with your arms or legs, you may find this activity to be too strenuous and should seek advice from your doctor or an experienced physical therapist.

Dangers of Stretching

Stretching is widely used throughout the world and most people believe it will do no harm. However, little research and evidence support the efficacy of stretching, and there are known dangers related to stretching.

Hypermobility, or the ability of a joint to move beyond the normal range of motion[45], increases the risk of injury. Sprains, strains and tears can occur by elongating, or stretching a muscle, beyond its normal capacity without building adequate strength. If a muscle does not have sufficient strength, then it can be injured with even the slightest movements or tasks.

Consistent stretching gives you excellent flexibility and mobility, but you must also make progress in strength training as well. Stretching is not a cure-all, nor will it give you perfect health. It may, however, enhance your quality of life and improve your daily activities and exercise routines. I further explain how to develop strength and flexibility together in _The 90-Day Home Workout Program_ and _The 3 Keys to Greater Health & Happiness_.

Basic Anatomy

It's important to know the areas that you are stretching when you use these exercises. Below are some basic diagrams of the areas you will feel the stretch most. Some stretches affect multiple sets of muscles. For simplicity's sake, I have narrowed down the primary muscle groups and areas that are affected. I've made the terminology simple.

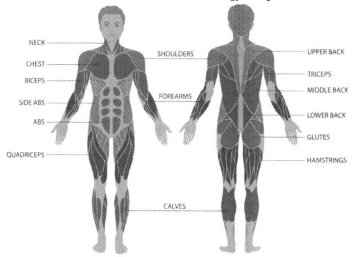

Other areas not pictured include:
- IT band – Located on the outer leg along the quadriceps
- Hip Flexors – Located on the front of the hip
- Inner Thighs (aka the groin)

Use this guide to help you figure out where you should feel a stretch, so it feels right. If you feel pain or discomfort in an area that is supposed to be benefited, stop immediately. Reassess your positioning and be sure that you are following the cues in each exercise to affect the proper area.

Stretch Programs

These stretch programs are developed with 2 different methods of a post-workout cool down and a standalone stretch routine. Go to the Glossary of Exercises after the exercise programs for exercise instructions (page 52). To help you become more familiar with an exercise, feel free to jot some notes in the lines below the exercise programs.

Each program has a unique set of exercises useful for a particular group of muscles. Whether isolating a muscle group in your workout or using a standalone stretch routine, I have a program for most needs.

Each workout has a distinct difficulty level. Easy is intended for anyone new to exercise. Intermediate is for someone experienced in exercise but has not consistently stretched. The advanced level is for experienced and conditioned athletes who need a challenge.

The difficulty levels are generalized suggestions and are not intended to be a substitute for your own judgment or for the recommendations of your doctor. Conduct every routine with caution, familiarize yourself with the entire routine before attempting and, most importantly, have fun doing the routines.

How to Get the Most from a Stretch

With all stretch exercises, get into position slowly and only go to a point of moderate tension. Causing excess discomfort or ignoring your pain threshold can negate any progress or results. If your body begins to shake or spasm, then you are stretching beyond your limitations. Perform a movement twice for the best results.

When stretching, pay close attention to how and where you most feel the stretch. Having mild discomfort in a stretch position is okay. If you continue to be uncomfortable after a stretch session, then you may be overstretching. The muscle or body part should not violently shake, spasm, or jitter in position. Stretch to the point that it feels uncomfortable, but not to a point that the muscle feels excessively tight and does not loosen up in the 6 to 30 seconds a stretch is applied. It takes 6 seconds to deactivate the stretch reflex, so that is the minimum time you need to use a functional stretch. There is no known benefit for holding a stretch for longer than 30 seconds, so limit your time holding any one stretch at a time.

Some quick guidelines to get the best stretch session include:

1) The muscle stretched must be free of any pre-existing conditions or injuries
2) A stretch should be applied only to the point of tension with mild discomfort, not pain
3) Ease into and out of all stretches, no exception
4) Never bounce in a stretch
5) Breathe in deeply before applying the stretch
6) Breathe out deliberately as you stretch
7) Consciously focus on relaxing the stretched muscle
8) Hold each stretch for 6-30 seconds each for the best results
9) Drink plenty of water after your stretch routine
10) Be sure to warm up before a stretch routine when advised. If you use a post-workout stretch program, then a warm-up may not be necessary.

Post Workout Routines

-10 minutes per routine

Lower Body Workouts

These programs are great for following up any lower body workout or activity.

Standing

Difficulty: Easy

	SIDE	EXERCISE	TIME	SETS
1	Left	Wall-Assisted Single Calf	20-30 sec.	2
2	Right	Wall-Assisted Single Calf	20-30 sec.	2
3	Left	Standing Hip Flexor	20-30 sec.	2
4	Right	Standing Hip Flexor	20-30 sec.	2
5	Left	Standing Ankle Pick	20-30 sec.	2
6	Right	Standing Ankle Pick	20-30 sec.	2
7	Left	Standing Bent Hamstring	20-30 sec.	2
8	Right	Standing Bent Hamstring	20-30 sec.	2
9	Left	Standing Cross-Legged Glute	20-30 sec.	2

NOTES:

_____

_____

_____

_____

_____

_____

_____

Seated to Lying

Difficulty: Easy

	SIDE	EXERCISE	TIME	SETS
1	Left	Seated Hamstring	20-30 sec.	2
2	Right	Seated Hamstring	20-30 sec.	2
3	Both	Seated Butterfly	20-30 sec.	2
4	Left	Seated Knee Hug	20-30 sec.	2
5	Right	Seated Knee Hug	20-30 sec.	2
6	Left	Seated Split-Leg Hamstring	20-30 sec.	2
7	Both	Knee Hug	20-30 sec.	2
8	Left	Lying Cross Leg Twist	20-30 sec.	2
9	Right	Lying Cross Leg Twist	20-30 sec.	2

NOTES:

_____

_____

_____

_____

_____

_____

_____

Kneeling to Seated

Difficulty: Easy to Intermediate

	SIDE	EXERCISE	TIME	SETS
1	Left	Kneeling Hip Flexor	20-30 sec.	2
2	Right	Kneeling Hip Flexor	20-30 sec.	2
3	Both	Kneeling Thigh	20-30 sec.	2
4	-	Kneeling Split Leg	20-30 sec.	2
5	Left	Seated Hamstring	20-30 sec.	2
6	Right	Seated Hamstring	20-30 sec.	2
7	Left	Pigeon Pose	20-30 sec.	2
8	Right	Pigeon Pose	20-30 sec.	2
9	Both	Child Pose	20-30 sec.	2

NOTES:

_____

_____

_____

_____

_____

_____

_____

Lying

Difficulty: Easy

	SIDE	EXERCISE	TIME	SETS
1	Left	Lying Hamstring	20-30 sec.	2
2	Right	Lying Hamstring	20-30 sec.	2
3	Left	Lying Figure-4	20-30 sec.	2
4	Right	Lying Figure-4	20-30 sec.	2
5	Both	Lying Butterfly	20-30 sec.	2
6	Left	Single Knee Hug	20-30 sec.	2
7	Right	Single Knee Hug	20-30 sec.	2
8	Left	Lying Cross Leg Twist	20-30 sec.	2
9	Right	Lying Cross Leg Twist	20-30 sec.	2
10	Both	Knee Hug	20-30 sec.	2

NOTES:

Hams, Hip Flexors, Inner Thighs, Calves
Difficulty: Easy to Intermediate

	SIDE	EXERCISE	TIME	SETS
1	Left	Deep Calf	20-30 sec.	2
2	Right	Deep Calf	20-30 sec.	2
3	Left	Strap Stretch: Bent Single Hamstring	20-30 sec.	2
4	Right	Strap Stretch: Bent Single Hamstring	20-30 sec.	2
5	Left	Kneeling Hip Flexor	20-30 sec.	2
6	Right	Kneeling Hip Flexor	20-30 sec.	2
7	Left	Strap Stretch: Seated Single Hamstring	20-30 sec.	2
8	Right	Strap Stretch: Seated Single Hamstring	20-30 sec.	2
9	Both	Strap Stretch: Seated Split-Leg Hamstring	20-30 sec.	2
10	Both	Seated Butterfly	20-30 sec.	2

NOTES:

_____

_____

_____

_____

_____

_____

_____

Total Hips I
Difficulty: Easy to Intermediate

	SIDE	EXERCISE	TIME	SETS
1	Left	Standing Hip Flexor	20-30 sec.	2
2	Right	Standing Hip Flexor	20-30 sec.	2
3	Left	Standing Cross-Legged Glute	20-30 sec.	2
4	Right	Standing Cross-Legged Glute	20-30 sec.	2
5	Left	Kneeling Hip Flexor	20-30 sec.	2
6	Right	Kneeling Hip Flexor	20-30 sec.	2
7	Both	Child Pose	20-30 sec.	2
8	Both	Cobra Pose	20-30 sec.	2
9	Left	Pigeon Pose	20-30 sec.	2
10	Right	Pigeon Pose	20-30 sec.	2

NOTES:

Upper Body Workouts

These programs are great for following up any upper body workout or activity.

Total Upper Body

Difficulty: Easy

	SIDE	EXERCISE	TIME	SETS
1	Left	Wall-Assisted Chest, Shoulder & Neck	20-30 sec.	2
2	Right	Wall-Assisted Chest, Shoulder & Neck	20-30 sec.	2
3	Both	Wall-Assisted Overhead Arm Hold	20-30 sec.	2
4	Both	Self Hug	20-30 sec.	2
5	Left	Single Shoulder/Elbow Grasp	20-30 sec.	2
6	Right	Single Shoulder/Elbow Grasp	20-30 sec.	2
7	Left	Forearm & Biceps Stretch	20-30 sec.	2
8	Right	Forearm & Biceps Stretch	20-30 sec.	2
9	Left	Forearm	20-30 sec.	2
10	Right	Forearm	20-30 sec.	2

NOTES:

Chest, Shoulders, Triceps, Neck

Difficulty: Easy to Intermediate

	SIDE	EXERCISE	TIME	SETS
1	Both	Strap Stretch: Chest & Shoulder	20-30 sec.	2
2	Left	Overhead Triceps	20-30 sec.	2
3	Right	Overhead Triceps	20-30 sec.	2
4	Left	Wall-Assisted Chest, Shoulder & Neck	20-30 sec.	2
5	Right	Wall-Assisted Chest, Shoulder & Neck	20-30 sec.	2
6	Left	Kneeling Shoulder & Back with Chair	20-30 sec.	2
7	Right	Kneeling Shoulder & Back with Chair	20-30 sec.	2
8	Both	Reverse Hug	20-30 sec.	2
9	-	Neck ROM (range-of-motion)	See instructions	2

NOTES:

_____

_____

_____

_____

_____

_____

_____

Back, Biceps, Forearms I
Difficulty: Easy to Intermediate

	SIDE	EXERCISE	TIME	SETS
1	Both	Self Hug	20-30 sec.	2
2	Both	Wall-Assisted Overhead Arm Hold	20-30 sec.	2
3	Left	Forearm & Biceps Stretch	20-30 sec.	2
4	Right	Forearm & Biceps Stretch	20-30 sec.	2
5	Both	Hanging Upper Body	20-30 sec.	2
6	Left	Wall-Assisted Straight Arm Chest, Shoulder & Neck	20-30 sec.	2
7	Right	Wall-Assisted Straight Arm Chest, Shoulder & Neck	20-30 sec.	2
8	Both	Hanging Upper Body	20-30 sec.	2
9	Left	Forearm	20-30 sec.	2
10	Right	Forearm	20-30 sec.	2

NOTES:

_____

_____

_____

_____

_____

_____

_____

Stand Alone Routines
-12 to 30 minutes per routine

Total Body Workout I
Difficulty: Intermediate to Advanced

	SIDE	EXERCISE	TIME	SETS
1	Both	Foam Roller: Back	~60 sec.	1
2	Left	Foam Roller: Single Glute	~60 sec.	1
3	Right	Foam Roller: Single Glute	~60 sec.	1
4	Left	Foam Roller: IT Band & Outer Thigh	~60 sec.	1
5	Right	Foam Roller: IT Band & Outer Thigh	~60 sec.	1
6	Both	Foam Roller: Hamstring	~60 sec.	1
7	Both	Foam Roller: Calves	~60 sec.	1
8	Both	Foam Roller: Hip Flexors	~60 sec.	1
9	-	Cat & Dog	~60 sec.	1
10	-	Child Pose	20-30 sec.	2
11	-	Cobra Pose	20-30 sec.	2
12	Left	Kneeling Hip Flexor	20-30 sec.	2
13	Right	Kneeling Hip Flexor	20-30 sec.	2
14	Left	Pigeon Pose	20-30 sec.	2
15	Right	Pigeon Pose	20-30 sec.	2
16	Left	Seated Hamstring	20-30 sec.	2
17	Right	Seated Hamstring	20-30 sec.	2
18	Left	Seated Knee Hug	20-30 sec.	2

19	Right	Seated Knee Hug	20-30 sec.	2
20	Both	Kneeling Shoulder & Back with Chair	20-30 sec.	2
21	Both	Overhead Interlaced Palms	20-30 sec.	2
22	Left	Wall-Assisted Chest, Shoulder & Neck	20-30 sec.	2
23	Right	Wall-Assisted Chest, Shoulder & Neck	20-30 sec.	2
24	Left	Overhead Triceps	20-30 sec.	2
25	Right	Overhead Triceps	20-30 sec.	2
26	Left	Rear Shoulder & Neck	20-30 sec.	2
27	Right	Rear Shoulder & Neck	20-30 sec.	2
28	Both	Self Hug	20-30 sec.	2
29	Both	Reverse Hug	20-30 sec.	2
30	-	Neck ROM (range-of-motion)	20-30 sec.	2

NOTES:

_____

_____

_____

_____

_____

_____

_____

Total Body Workout II

Difficulty: Intermediate to Advanced

	SIDE	EXERCISE	TIME	SETS
1	Both	Foam Roller: Back	~60 sec.	1
2	Left	Foam Roller: Side Lying Back	~60 sec.	1
3	Right	Foam Roller: Side Lying Back	~60 sec.	1
4	Left	Foam Roller: Single Hip Flexor	~60 sec.	1
5	Right	Foam Roller: Single Hip Flexor	~60 sec.	1
6	Left	Foam Roller: IT Band & Outer Thigh	~60 sec.	1
7	Right	Foam Roller: IT Band & Outer Thigh	~60 sec.	1
8	Both	Foam Roller: Hamstring	~60 sec.	1
9	Left	Foam Roller: Outer Calf	~60 sec.	1
10	Right	Foam Roller: Outer Calf	~60 sec.	1
11	Both	Kneeling Thigh	20-30 sec.	2
12	Both	Kneeling Split Leg	20-30 sec.	2
13	Left	Child Pose with Arm Thread	20-30 sec.	2
14	Right	Child Pose with Arm Thread	20-30 sec.	2
15	Both	Kneeling Shoulder & Back with Chair	20-30 sec.	2
16	Left	Overhead Triceps	20-30 sec.	2
17	Right	Overhead Triceps	20-30 sec.	2
18	Left	Side Lying Ankle Pick	20-30 sec.	2
19	Right	Side Lying Ankle Pick	20-30 sec.	2

20	Left	Lying Figure-4	20-30 sec.	2
21	Right	Lying Figure-4	20-30 sec.	2
22	Left	Strap Stretch: Lying Hamstring	20-30 sec.	2
23	Right	Strap Stretch: Lying Hamstring	20-30 sec.	2
24	Left	Strap Stretch: Iron Cross	20-30 sec.	2
25	Right	Strap Stretch: Iron Cross	20-30 sec.	2
26	Both	Overhead Interlaced Palms	20-30 sec.	2
27	Left	Single Shoulder/Elbow Grasp	20-30 sec.	2
28	Right	Single Shoulder/Elbow Grasp	20-30 sec.	2
29	Left	Wall-Assisted Chest, Shoulder & Neck	20-30 sec.	2
30	Right	Wall-Assisted Chest, Shoulder & Neck	20-30 sec.	2

NOTES:

_____

_____

_____

_____

_____

_____

_____

Total Body Workout III

Difficulty: Intermediate to Advanced

	SIDE	EXERCISE	TIME	SETS
1	Both	Foam Roller: Calves	~60 sec.	1
2	Left	Foam Roller: Outer Calf	~60 sec.	1
3	Right	Foam Roller: Outer Calf	~60 sec.	1
4	Left	Foam Roller: Single Hamstring	~60 sec.	1
5	Right	Foam Roller: Single Hamstring	~60 sec.	1
6	Left	Foam Roller: IT Band & Outer Thigh	~60 sec.	1
7	Right	Foam Roller: IT Band & Outer Thigh	~60 sec.	1
8	Left	Foam Roller: Single Glute	~60 sec.	1
9	Right	Foam Roller: Single Glute	~60 sec.	1
10	Both	Foam Roller: Back	~60 sec.	1
11	Left	Wall-Assisted Single Leg Hamstring	20-30 sec.	2
12	Right	Wall-Assisted Single Leg Hamstring	20-30 sec.	2
13	Both	Wall-Assisted Butterfly	20-30 sec.	2
14	Both	Wall-Assisted Lying Split-Leg Hamstring	20-30 sec.	2
15	Both	Child Pose	20-30 sec.	2
16	Both	Cobra Pose	20-30 sec.	2
17	Left	Pigeon Pose	20-30 sec.	2
18	Right	Pigeon Pose	20-30 sec.	2

19	Left	Kneeling Hip Flexor	20-30 sec.	2
20	Right	Kneeling Hip Flexor	20-30 sec.	2
21	Both	Overhead Interlaced Palms	20-30 sec.	2
22	Left	Forearm & Biceps Stretch	20-30 sec.	2
23	Right	Forearm & Biceps Stretch	20-30 sec.	2
24	Both	Strap Stretch: Chest & Shoulder	20-30 sec.	2
25	Left	Strap Stretch: Overhead Triceps	20-30 sec.	2
26	Right	Strap Stretch: Overhead Triceps	20-30 sec.	2
27	Both	Wall-Assisted Overhead Arm Hold	20-30 sec.	2
28	Left	Rear Shoulder & Neck	20-30 sec.	2
29	Right	Rear Shoulder & Neck	20-30 sec.	2
30	-	Neck ROM (range-of-motion)	20-30 sec.	2

NOTES:

_____

_____

_____

_____

_____

_____

Total Body Workout IV

Difficulty: Intermediate to Advanced

	SIDE	EXERCISE	TIME	SETS
1	Both	Foam Roller: Hip Flexors	~60 sec.	1
2	Left	Foam Roller: Single Hip Flexor	~60 sec.	1
3	Right	Foam Roller: Single Hip Flexor	~60 sec.	1
4	Left	Foam Roller: Side Lying Back	~60 sec.	1
5	Right	Foam Roller: Side Lying Back	~60 sec.	1
6	Both	Foam Roller: Back	~60 sec.	1
7	Left	Foam Roller: Single Hamstring	~60 sec.	1
8	Right	Foam Roller: Single Hamstring	~60 sec.	1
9	Left	Foam Roller: IT Band & Outer Thigh	~60 sec.	1
10	Right	Foam Roller: IT Band & Outer Thigh	~60 sec.	1
11	-	Neck ROM (range-of-motion)	20-30 sec.	2
12	Both	Overhead Interlaced Palms	20-30 sec.	2
13	-	Wall-Assisted Overhead Arm Hold	20-30 sec.	2
14	Left	Wall-Assisted Straight Arm Chest, Shoulder & Neck	20-30 sec.	2
15	Right	Wall-Assisted Straight Arm Chest, Shoulder & Neck	20-30 sec.	2
16	Left	Overhead Triceps	20-30 sec.	2
17	Right	Overhead Triceps	20-30 sec.	2
18	Both	Self Hug	20-30 sec.	2

19	Both	Reverse Hug	20-30 sec.	2
20	Left	Standing Ankle Pick	20-30 sec.	2
21	Right	Standing Ankle Pick	20-30 sec.	2
22	Left	Standing Hip Flexor	20-30 sec.	2
23	Right	Standing Hip Flexor	20-30 sec.	2
24	Left	Standing Bent Hamstring	20-30 sec.	2
25	Right	Standing Bent Hamstring	20-30 sec.	2
26	Left	Standing Cross-Legged Glute	20-30 sec.	2
27	Right	Standing Cross-Legged Glute	20-30 sec.	2
28	Left	Deep Calf	20-30 sec.	2
29	Right	Deep Calf	20-30 sec.	2

NOTES:

_____

_____

_____

_____

_____

_____

_____

_____

_____

Lower Body Workout

Difficulty: Intermediate to Advanced

	SIDE	EXERCISE	TIME	SETS
1	Both	Foam Roller: Back	~60 sec.	1
2	Left	Foam Roller: Single Glute	~60 sec.	1
3	Right	Foam Roller: Single Glute	~60 sec.	1
4	Left	Foam Roller: IT Band & Outer Thigh	~60 sec.	1
5	Right	Foam Roller: IT Band & Outer Thigh	~60 sec.	1
6	Both	Foam Roller: Hamstring	~60 sec.	1
7	Both	Foam Roller: Calves	~60 sec.	1
8	Both	Foam Roller: Hip Flexors	~60 sec.	1
9	-	Cat & Dog	~60 sec.	1
10	-	Child Pose	20-30 sec.	2
11	-	Cobra Pose	20-30 sec.	2
12	Left	Single Calf (pike)	20-30 sec.	2
13	Right	Single Calf (pike)	20-30 sec.	2
14	Left	Kneeling Hip Flexor	20-30 sec.	2
15	Right	Kneeling Hip Flexor	20-30 sec.	2
16	Left	Pigeon Pose	20-30 sec.	2
17	Right	Pigeon Pose	20-30 sec.	2
18	Left	Side Lying Ankle Pick	20-30 sec.	2
19	Right	Side Lying Ankle Pick	20-30 sec.	2

20	Both	Seated Hamstring	20-30 sec.	2
21	Both	Seated Hamstring	20-30 sec.	2
22	Left	Seated Knee Hug	20-30 sec.	2
23	Right	Seated Knee Hug	20-30 sec.	2
24	Left	Seated Butterfly	20-30 sec.	2
25	Right	Seated Split-Leg Hamstring	20-30 sec.	2
26	Left	Strap Stretch: Lying Hamstring	20-30 sec.	2
27	Right	Strap Stretch: Lying Hamstring	20-30 sec.	2
28	Left	Strap Stretch: Lying Figure Four	20-30 sec.	2
29	Right	Strap Stretch: Lying Figure Four	20-30 sec.	2
30	Both	Knee Hug	20-30 sec.	2

NOTES:

_____

_____

_____

_____

_____

_____

_____

_____

Hams, Hip Flexors, Calves

Difficulty: Intermediate to Advanced

	SIDE	EXERCISE	TIME	SETS
1	Both	Foam Roller: Calves	~60 sec.	1
2	Left	Foam Roller: Single Calf	~60 sec.	1
3	Right	Foam Roller: Single Calf	~60 sec.	1
4	Both	Foam Roller: Hamstring	~60 sec.	1
5	Left	Foam Roller: Single Hamstring	~60 sec.	1
6	Right	Foam Roller: Single Hamstring	~60 sec.	1
7	Both	Foam Roller: Hip Flexors	~60 sec.	1
8	Left	Foam Roller: Single Hip Flexor	~60 sec.	1
9	Right	Foam Roller: Single Hip Flexor	~60 sec.	1
10	Left	Strap Stretch: Lying Hamstring	20-30 sec.	2
11	Right	Strap Stretch: Lying Hamstring	20-30 sec.	2
12	Left	Strap Stretch: Side Lying Thigh & Hip Flexor	20-30 sec.	2
13	Right	Strap Stretch: Side Lying Thigh & Hip Flexor	20-30 sec.	2
14	Left	Single Calf (pike)	20-30 sec.	2
15	Right	Single Calf (pike)	20-30 sec.	2
16	Left	Kneeling Hip Flexor	20-30 sec.	2
17	Right	Kneeling Hip Flexor	20-30 sec.	2
18	Left	Standing Bent Hamstring	20-30 sec.	2
19	Right	Standing Bent Hamstring	20-30 sec.	2

20	Left	Step Assisted Single Calf	20-30 sec.	2
21	Right	Step Assisted Single Calf	20-30 sec.	2
22	Left	Standing Hip Flexor	20-30 sec.	2
23	Right	Standing Hip Flexor	20-30 sec.	2
24	Left	Standing Elevated Hamstring	20-30 sec.	2
25	Right	Standing Elevated Hamstring	20-30 sec.	2
26	Left	Deep Calf	20-30 sec.	2
27	Right	Deep Calf	20-30 sec.	2

NOTES:

_____

_____

_____

_____

_____

_____

_____

_____

_____

_____

_____

Total Hips II

Difficulty: Intermediate to Advanced
Warm-up 5-10 minutes before this routine for best results

	SIDE	EXERCISE	TIME	SETS
1	Left	Foam Roller: Single Glute	~60 sec.	1
2	Right	Foam Roller: Single Glute	~60 sec.	1
3	Both	Foam Roller: Hip Flexors	~60 sec.	1
4	Left	Foam Roller: Single Hip Flexor	~60 sec.	1
5	Right	Foam Roller: Single Hip Flexor	~60 sec.	1
6	Both	Knee Hug	20-30 sec.	2
7	Left	Strap Stretch: Lying Figure Four	20-30 sec.	2
8	Right	Strap Stretch: Lying Figure Four	20-30 sec.	2
9	Left	Strap Stretch: Lying Single Thigh	20-30 sec.	2
10	Right	Strap Stretch: Lying Single Thigh	20-30 sec.	2
11	Left	Strap Stretch: Side Lying Thigh & Hip Flexor	20-30 sec.	2
12	Right	Strap Stretch: Side Lying Thigh & Hip Flexor	20-30 sec.	2
13	Left	Seated Knee Hug	20-30 sec.	2
14	Right	Seated Knee Hug	20-30 sec.	2
15	Left	Kneeling Hip Flexor	20-30 sec.	2
16	Right	Kneeling Hip Flexor	20-30 sec.	2
17	Left	Pigeon Pose	20-30 sec.	2

18	Right	Pigeon Pose	20-30 sec.	2
19	Left	Standing Hip Flexor	20-30 sec.	2
20	Right	Standing Hip Flexor	20-30 sec.	2
21	Left	Standing Cross-Legged Glute	20-30 sec.	2
22	Right	Standing Cross-Legged Glute	20-30 sec.	2
23	Left	Child Pose	20-30 sec.	2
24	Right	Cobra Pose	20-30 sec.	2

NOTES:

_____

_____

_____

_____

_____

_____

_____

_____

_____

_____

_____

Upper Body Workouts

Difficulty: Intermediate to Advanced
Warm-up 6-10 minutes before this routine for best results

	SIDE	EXERCISE	TIME	SETS
1	Both	Foam Roller: Back	~60 sec.	1
2	Left	Foam Roller: Side Lying Back	~60 sec.	1
3	Right	Foam Roller: Side Lying Back	~60 sec.	1
4	Both	Cat & Dog	~60 sec.	1
5	Left	Child Pose with Arm Thread	20-30 sec.	2
6	Right	Child Pose with Arm Thread	20-30 sec.	2
7	Both	Cobra Pose	20-30 sec.	2
8	Both	Hanging Upper Body	20-30 sec.	2
9	Both	Strap Stretch: Chest & Shoulder	20-30 sec.	2
10	Left	Wall-Assisted Straight Arm Chest, Shoulder & Neck	20-30 sec.	2
11	Right	Wall-Assisted Straight Arm Chest, Shoulder & Neck	20-30 sec.	2
12	Both	Overhead Interlaced Palms	20-30 sec.	2
13	Both	Wall-Assisted Overhead Arm Hold	20-30 sec.	2
14	Both	Hanging Upper Body	20-30 sec.	2
15	Left	Forearm & Biceps Stretch	20-30 sec.	2

16	Right	Forearm & Biceps Stretch	20-30 sec.	2
17	Left	Forearm	20-30 sec.	2
18	Right	Forearm	20-30 sec.	2
19	Left	Wall-Assisted Chest, Shoulder & Neck	20-30 sec.	2
20	Right	Wall-Assisted Chest, Shoulder & Neck	20-30 sec.	2
21	Left	Strap Stretch: Overhead Triceps	20-30 sec.	2
22	Right	Strap Stretch: Overhead Triceps	20-30 sec.	2
23	Left	Rear Shoulder & Neck	20-30 sec.	2
24	Right	Rear Shoulder & Neck	20-30 sec.	2
25	Both	Self Hug	20-30 sec.	2
26	Both	Reverse Hug	20-30 sec.	2
27	Both	Neck ROM (range-of-motion)	20-30 sec.	2

NOTES:

_____

_____

_____

_____

_____

Chest, Shoulders, Neck

Difficulty: Easy to Intermediate
Warm-up 10 minutes before this routine for best results

	SIDE	EXERCISE	TIME	SETS
1	-	Child Pose	20-30 sec.	2
2	-	Cobra Pose	20-30 sec.	2
3	Left	Kneeling Shoulder & Back with Chair	20-30 sec.	2
4	Right	Overhead Interlaced Palms	20-30 sec.	2
5	Left	Wall-Assisted Chest, Shoulder & Neck	20-30 sec.	2
6	Right	Wall-Assisted Chest, Shoulder & Neck	20-30 sec.	2
7	Left	Rear Shoulder & Neck	20-30 sec.	2
8	Right	Rear Shoulder & Neck	20-30 sec.	2
9	Left	Single Shoulder/Elbow Grasp	20-30 sec.	2
10	Right	Single Shoulder/Elbow Grasp	20-30 sec.	2
11	Both	Strap Stretch: Chest & Shoulder	20-30 sec.	2
12	Both	Self Hug	20-30 sec.	2
13	Both	Reverse Hug	20-30 sec.	2
14	-	Neck ROM (range-of-motion)	20-30 sec.	2

NOTES:

Back, Biceps, Forearms II

Difficulty: Intermediate to Advanced
Warm-up 7-10 minutes before this routine for best results

	SIDE	EXERCISE	TIME	SETS
1	Both	Foam Roller: Back	~60 sec.	1
2	Left	Foam Roller: Side Lying Back	~60 sec.	1
3	Right	Foam Roller: Side Lying Back	~60 sec.	1
4	Left	Child Pose with Arm Thread	~60 sec.	1
5	Right	Child Pose with Arm Thread	~60 sec.	1
6	Both	Kneeling Shoulder & Back with Chair	~60 sec.	1
7	Left	Wall-Assisted Straight Arm Chest, Shoulder & Neck	~60 sec.	1
8	Right	Wall-Assisted Straight Arm Chest, Shoulder & Neck	~60 sec.	1
9	Both	Hanging Upper Body	20-30 sec.	2
10	Both	Wall-Assisted Overhead Arm Hold	20-30 sec.	2
11	Left	Forearm & Biceps Stretch	20-30 sec.	2
12	Right	Forearm & Biceps Stretch	20-30 sec.	2
13	Left	Overhead Interlaced Palms	20-30 sec.	2
14	Right	Forearm	20-30 sec.	2
15	Left	Forearm	20-30 sec.	2

NOTES:

_____

_____

_____

Chest, Triceps, Forearms

Difficulty: Easy to Intermediate
Warm-up 10 minutes before this routine for best results

	SIDE	EXERCISE	TIME	SETS
1	Left	Wall-Assisted Chest, Shoulder & Neck	20-30 sec.	2
2	Right	Wall-Assisted Chest, Shoulder & Neck	20-30 sec.	2
3	Both	Overhead Interlaced Palms	20-30 sec.	2
4	Left	Strap Stretch: Overhead Triceps	20-30 sec.	2
5	Right	Strap Stretch: Overhead Triceps	20-30 sec.	2
6	Both	Strap Stretch: Chest & Shoulder	20-30 sec.	2
7	Left	Rear Shoulder & Neck	20-30 sec.	2
8	Right	Rear Shoulder & Neck	20-30 sec.	2
9	Left	Forearm	20-30 sec.	2
10	Right	Forearm	20-30 sec.	2
11	Left	Single Shoulder/Elbow Grasp	20-30 sec.	2
12	Right	Single Shoulder/Elbow Grasp	20-30 sec.	2
13	-	Reverse Hug	20-30 sec.	2

NOTES:

Seated Exclusive

Difficulty: Easy
Warm-up 10 minutes before this routine for best results

	SIDE	EXERCISE	TIME	SETS
1	Left	Seated Hamstring	20-30 sec.	2
2	Right	Seated Hamstring	20-30 sec.	2
3	Both	Seated Butterfly	20-30 sec.	2
4	Left	Seated Split-Leg Hamstring	20-30 sec.	2
5	Left	Seated Knee Hug	20-30 sec.	2
6	Right	Seated Knee Hug	20-30 sec.	2
7	Left	Single Shoulder/Elbow Grasp	20-30 sec.	2
8	Right	Single Shoulder/Elbow Grasp	20-30 sec.	2
9	Both	Overhead Interlaced Palms	20-30 sec.	2
10	Left	Overhead Triceps	20-30 sec.	2
11	Right	Overhead Triceps	20-30 sec.	2
12	Left	Forearm	20-30 sec.	2
13	Right	Forearm	20-30 sec.	2
14	Left	Rear Shoulder & Neck	20-30 sec.	2
15	Right	Rear Shoulder & Neck	20-30 sec.	2
16	Both	Self Hug	20-30 sec.	2
17	Both	Reverse Hug	20-30 sec.	2
18	Both	Neck ROM (range-of-motion)	20-30 sec.	2

NOTES:

Standing Exclusive

Difficulty: Easy
Warm-up 10 minutes before this routine for best results

	SIDE	EXERCISE	TIME	SETS
1	Left	Step Assisted Single Calf	20-30 sec.	2
2	Right	Step Assisted Single Calf	20-30 sec.	2
3	Left	Standing Ankle Pick	20-30 sec.	2
4	Right	Standing Ankle Pick	20-30 sec.	2
5	Left	Standing Hip Flexor	20-30 sec.	2
6	Right	Standing Hip Flexor	20-30 sec.	2
7	Left	Standing Cross-Legged Glute	20-30 sec.	2
8	Right	Standing Cross-Legged Glute	20-30 sec.	2
9	Left	Standing Elevated Hamstring	20-30 sec.	2
10	Right	Standing Elevated Hamstring	20-30 sec.	2
11	Left	Wall-Assisted Chest, Shoulder & Neck	20-30 sec.	2
12	Right	Wall-Assisted Chest, Shoulder & Neck	20-30 sec.	2
13	Both	Wall-Assisted Overhead Arm Hold	20-30 sec.	2
14	Both	Hanging Upper Body	20-30 sec.	2
15	Left	Single Shoulder/Elbow Grasp	20-30 sec.	2
16	Right	Single Shoulder/Elbow Grasp	20-30 sec.	2
17	Left	Lateral Leg	20-30 sec.	2
18	Right	Lateral Leg	20-30 sec.	2
19	Left	Forearm	20-30 sec.	2

20	Right	Forearm	20-30 sec.	2
21	Both	Overhead Interlaced Palms	20-30 sec.	2
22	Left	Forearm & Biceps Stretch	20-30 sec.	2
23	Right	Forearm & Biceps Stretch	20-30 sec.	2
24	Left	Overhead Triceps	20-30 sec.	2
25	Right	Overhead Triceps	20-30 sec.	2
26	Left	Rear Shoulder & Neck	20-30 sec.	2
27	Right	Rear Shoulder & Neck	20-30 sec.	2
28	Both	Self Hug	20-30 sec.	2
29	Both	Reverse Hug	20-30 sec.	2
30	Both	Neck ROM (range-of-motion)	20-30 sec.	2

NOTES:

_____

_____

_____

_____

_____

_____

_____

_____

_____

Kneeling Exclusive

Difficulty: Easy to Intermediate
Warm-up 10 minutes before this routine for best results

	SIDE	EXERCISE	TIME	SETS
1	-	Cat & Dog	~60 sec.	1
2	Both	Kneeling Thigh	20-30 sec.	2
3	-	Child Pose	20-30 sec.	2
4	-	Cobra Pose	20-30 sec.	2
5	Left	Kneeling Hip Flexor	20-30 sec.	2
6	Right	Kneeling Hip Flexor	20-30 sec.	2
7	Left	Pigeon Pose	20-30 sec.	2
8	Right	Pigeon Pose	20-30 sec.	2
9	Both	Kneeling Split Leg	20-30 sec.	2
10	Both	Kneeling Shoulder & Back with Chair	20-30 sec.	2
11	Left	Child Pose with Arm Thread	20-30 sec.	2
12	Right	Child Pose with Arm Thread	20-30 sec.	2

NOTES:

_____

_____

_____

_____

_____

_____

_____

Sedentary Worker

Difficulty: Easy to Intermediate
Warm-up 10 minutes before this routine for best results

	SIDE	EXERCISE	TIME	SETS
1	Left	Wall-Assisted Single Calf	20-30 sec.	2
2	Right	Wall-Assisted Single Calf	20-30 sec.	2
3	Left	Deep Calf	20-30 sec.	2
4	Right	Deep Calf	20-30 sec.	2
5	Left	Standing Hip Flexor	20-30 sec.	2
6	Right	Standing Hip Flexor	20-30 sec.	2
7	Left	Standing Elevated Hamstring	20-30 sec.	2
8	Right	Standing Elevated Hamstring	20-30 sec.	2
9	Left	Standing Cross-Legged Glute	20-30 sec.	2
10	Right	Standing Cross-Legged Glute	20-30 sec.	2
11	Left	Kneeling Hip Flexor	20-30 sec.	2
12	Right	Kneeling Hip Flexor	20-30 sec.	2
13	Both	Kneeling Thigh	20-30 sec.	2
14	-	Child Pose	20-30 sec.	2
15	-	Cobra Pose	20-30 sec.	2
16	Left	Pigeon Pose	20-30 sec.	2
17	Right	Pigeon Pose	20-30 sec.	2
18	-	Neck ROM (range-of-motion)	20-30 sec.	2
19	Left	Forearm	20-30 sec.	2
20	Right	Forearm	20-30 sec.	2

21	-	Overhead Interlaced Palms	20-30 sec.	2
22	Left	Forearm & Biceps Stretch	20-30 sec.	2
23	Right	Forearm & Biceps Stretch	20-30 sec.	2
24	Left	Wall-Assisted Chest, Shoulder & Neck	20-30 sec.	2
25	Right	Wall-Assisted Chest, Shoulder & Neck	20-30 sec.	2
26	Left	Rear Shoulder & Neck	20-30 sec.	2
27	Right	Rear Shoulder & Neck	20-30 sec.	2
28	Both	Strap Stretch: Chest & Shoulder	20-30 sec.	2
29	Left	Single Shoulder/Elbow Grasp	20-30 sec.	2
30	Right	Single Shoulder/Elbow Grasp	20-30 sec.	2

NOTES:

_____

_____

_____

_____

_____

_____

_____

_____

Strap Stretch

Difficulty: Easy to Intermediate
Warm-up 10 minutes before this routine for best results

	SIDE	EXERCISE	TIME	SETS
1	Left	Strap Stretch: Bent Single Hamstring	20-30 sec.	2
2	Right	Strap Stretch: Bent Single Hamstring	20-30 sec.	2
3	Both	Strap Stretch: Chest & Shoulder	20-30 sec.	2
4	Left	Strap Stretch: Overhead Triceps	20-30 sec.	2
5	Right	Strap Stretch: Overhead Triceps	20-30 sec.	2
6	Left	Strap Stretch: Seated Single Hamstring	20-30 sec.	2
7	Right	Strap Stretch: Seated Single Hamstring	20-30 sec.	2
8	-	Strap Stretch: Seated Split-Leg Hamstring	20-30 sec.	2
9	Left	Strap Stretch: Lying Single Thigh	20-30 sec.	2
10	Right	Strap Stretch: Lying Single Thigh	20-30 sec.	2
11	Left	Strap Stretch: Lying Hamstring	20-30 sec.	2
12	Right	Strap Stretch: Lying Hamstring	20-30 sec.	2
13	Left	Strap Stretch: Lying Figure Four	20-30 sec.	2
14	Right	Strap Stretch: Lying Figure Four	20-30 sec.	2

15	Left	Strap Stretch: Iron Cross	20-30 sec.	2
16	Right	Strap Stretch: Iron Cross	20-30 sec.	2
17	Left	Strap Stretch: Side Lying Thigh & Hip Flexor	20-30 sec.	2
18	Right	Strap Stretch: Side Lying Thigh & Hip Flexor	20-30 sec.	2

NOTES:

_____

_____

_____

_____

_____

_____

_____

_____

_____

_____

_____

_____

Foam Rolling

Difficulty: Intermediate to Advanced

	SIDE	EXERCISE	TIME	SETS
1	Both	Foam Roller: Back	~60 sec.	1
2	Left	Foam Roller: Side Lying Back	~60 sec.	1
3	Right	Foam Roller: Side Lying Back	~60 sec.	1
4	Left	Foam Roller: Single Glute	~60 sec.	1
5	Right	Foam Roller: Single Glute	~60 sec.	1
6	Left	Foam Roller: IT Band & Outer Thigh	~60 sec.	1
7	Right	Foam Roller: IT Band & Outer Thigh	~60 sec.	1
8	Both	Foam Roller: Hip Flexors	~60 sec.	1
9	Left	Foam Roller: Single Hip Flexor	~60 sec.	1
10	Right	Foam Roller: Single Hip Flexor	~60 sec.	1
11	Both	Foam Roller: Hamstring	~60 sec.	1
12	Left	Foam Roller: Single Hamstring	~60 sec.	1
13	Right	Foam Roller: Single Hamstring	~60 sec.	1
14	Both	Foam Roller: Calves	~60 sec.	1
15	Left	Foam Roller: Outer Calf	~60 sec.	1
16	Right	Foam Roller: Outer Calf	~60 sec.	1

NOTES:

_____

_____

_____

Glossary of Stretches

Cat & Dog
Affects: lower back, neck

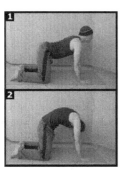

From a kneeling position, place your palms below your shoulders. Arch your spine upward and look toward your knees. Relax from the position, push your spine downward and then lift your chin upward. Hold each position for half the usual stretch time.

Related programs: Total Body Workout I, Lower Body Workout, Upper Body Workouts, Kneeling Exclusive

Child Pose
Affects: glutes, upper back, middle back, thighs

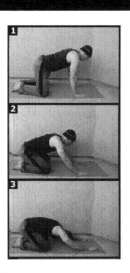

Kneel down on the floor, and place your glutes on your heels. Slowly bring your stomach to your thighs, your chest to the floor and extend your arms out above your head.

Related programs: Kneeling to Seated, Total Hips I, Total Body Workout I, Total Body Workout III, Lower Body Workout, Total Hips II, Chest, Shoulders, Neck, Kneeling Exclusive, Sedentary Worker

Child Pose with Arm Thread

Affects: glutes, upper back, middle back, thighs

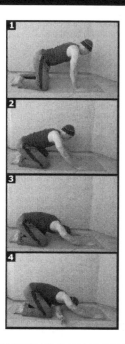

Kneel down on the floor, and place your glutes on your heels. Slowly bring your stomach to your thighs, your chest to the floor and extend your arms out above your head. Then, insert one arm under and across your chest.

Related programs: Total Body Workout II, Upper Body Workouts, Back, Biceps, Forearms II, Kneeling Exclusive

Cobra Pose

Affects: hip flexors, abs, neck

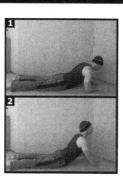

Lie on your stomach with your elbows bent below your shoulders and your palms placed on the floor. Extend your arms and arch your spine upward while lifting your chin.

Related programs: Total Hips I, Total Body Workout I, Total Body Workout III, Lower Body Workout, Total Hips II, Upper Body Workouts, Chest, Shoulders, Neck, Kneeling Exclusive, Sedentary Worker

Deep Calf
Affects: calves

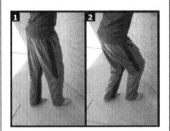

Stand one to two steps away from the wall. Place your palms on the wall with your arms slightly extended. Separate your stance about hip-width apart. Bring one foot closer to the wall and then bring the back foot behind front foot. Bend both knees, and sink into the heels while lifting both big toes. If you do not feel a stretch, then step further away from the wall, and try again. To feel a deeper stretch, drop your butt to the ground more.

Related programs: Hams, Hip Flexors, Inner Thighs, Calves, Total Body Workout IV, Hams, Hip Flexors, Calves, Sedentary Worker

Foam Roller: Back
Affects: middle back, upper back

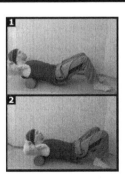

Start with the foam roller placed below your mid-back. Bend your knees and keep your feet flat on the floor. Support your head with your hands. Pick your butt off the floor. Draw your butt toward your heels and foam roll up to just below your shoulders. Then, move the opposite direction toward your low back and stop just short of your low back.

Related programs: Total Body Workout I, Total Body Workout II, Total Body Workout III, Total Body Workout IV, Lower Body Workout, Upper Body Workouts, Back, Biceps, Forearms II, Foam Rolling

Foam Roller: Calves
Affects: calves

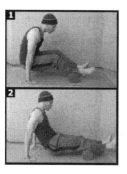

Sit on the floor and place the foam roller under the middle of your calves. Put your hands on the ground behind you to support your weight. Roll up and down the calf between your ankle and below your knee.

Related programs: Total Body Workout I, Total Body Workout III, Lower Body Workout, Hams, Hip Flexors, Calves, Foam Rolling

Foam Roller: Hamstring
Affects: hamstrings

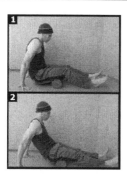

Sit on the floor and place the foam roller under the middle of your hamstrings. Put your hands on the ground behind you to support your weight. Roll up and down the back of your thighs between your butt and above your knee.

Related programs: Total Body Workout I, Total Body Workout II, Lower Body Workout, Hams, Hip Flexors, Calves, Foam Rolling

Helpful Tip: Focus on breathing naturally when using the foam roller. Foam rolling can be physically demanding so it will take practice and patience.

Foam Roller: Hip Flexors
Affects: hip flexors

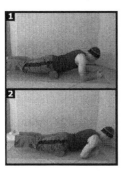

Lie face down with the foam roller below the front of your hip. Support your upper body with your forearms and elbows. Roll above your hips and down into the top of your thighs.

Related programs: Total Body Workout I, Total Body Workout IV, Lower Body Workout, Hams, Hip Flexors, Calves, Total Hips II, Foam Rolling

Foam Roller: IT Band & Outer Thigh
Affects: IT band, outer quadriceps

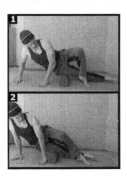

Lie on your side with the foam roller under your middle of your bottom leg. Roll from the lower part of your hip to above your knee.

Related programs: Total Body Workout I, Total Body Workout II, Total Body Workout III, Total Body Workout IV, Lower Body Workout, Foam Rolling

---

Helpful Tip: Foam rolling requires a little trial and error in placement. If you feel nothing, then you may have to adjust the placement. However, if you get any discomfort, then you may have hit the right area. Try to roll carefully and ease your weight over the tight area.

Foam Roller: Outer Calf
Affects: outer calf

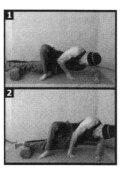

Lie on your side with the foam roller under your bottom leg at the middle of the calf. Roll from below your knee to above your ankle.

Related programs: Total Body Workout II, Total Body Workout III, Foam Rolling

Foam Roller: Side Lying Back
Affects: outer-middle back

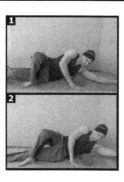

Lie on your side with the foam roller around the middle of your ribs. Roll from below your armpit to above the bottom of your ribs.

Related programs: Total Body Workout II, Total Body Workout IV, Upper Body Workouts, Back, Biceps, Forearms II, Foam Rolling

Helpful Tip: A variety of foam rollers are on the market these days. Start with a medium-density foam roller. Once you master using it, graduate to a thicker density. Avoid the fancy foam rollers with the ridges, bumps and extra bells and whistles. Those are neat, but not necessary for beginners.

Foam Roller: Single Calf
Affects: calf

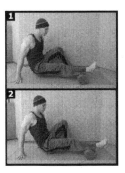

Sit on the floor and place the foam roller under only one leg at the middle of your calf. Bend the other leg and place your foot flat on the floor. Put your hands behind you to support your weight. Roll up and down the calf between your ankle and knee.

Related programs: Hams, Hip Flexors, Calves

Foam Roller: Single Glute
Affects: glutes

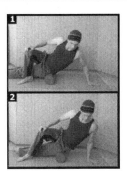

Sit on the foam roller and angle your body to one side. Place the roller between your hip bone and your tailbone. Roll up and down over your glutes on one side. Foam roll each side equally.

Related programs: Total Body Workout I, Total Body Workout III, Lower Body Workout, Total Hips II, Foam Rolling

Fun Fact: Areas commonly with knots are the glutes, IT bands, outer calves. Roll those areas before a workout session to get the most from your exercises.

Foam Roller: Single Hamstring
Affects: hamstrings

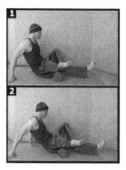

Sit on the floor and place the foam roller under the middle of your thigh. Bend the other knee and cross your foot over your thigh. Use your hands behind you to support your weight. Roll up and down your hamstrings between your butt and above your knee. Foam roll each side equally.

Related programs: Total Body Workout III, Total Body Workout IV, Hams, Hip Flexors, Calves, Foam Rolling

Foam Roller: Single Hip Flexor
Affects: hip flexors

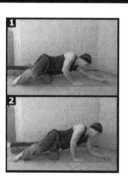

Lie face down, slightly to the side with the foam roller at the front of one hip. Bend the other leg and place your foot on the ground. Support your upper body with your forearms and elbows. Roll above your hips and down into the top of your thighs. Foam roll each side equally.

Related programs: Total Body Workout II, Total Body Workout IV, Hams, Hip Flexors, Calves, Total Hips II, Foam Rolling

Helpful Tip: Clear out plenty of space for foam rolling, so you are uninhibited in your movements.

Forearm

Affects: forearm, wrist

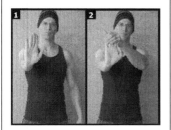

Extend one arm in front of you with your palm faced away from your body and fingers pointed up. Grasp your fingertips and pull back with your free hand.

Related programs: Back, Biceps, Forearms I, Total Upper Body, Back, Biceps, Forearms II, Upper Body Workouts

Forearm & Biceps Stretch

Affects: forearm, biceps, wrist

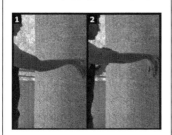

Step within arm's reach of the wall. With your arm extended out and your palm faced up below shoulder level, slowly flatten your palm against the wall. Keep your fingers pointed down and the inside of your elbow turned up. If this stretch is new to you, then start with your hand lower on the wall for less tension.

Related programs: Total Upper Body, Back, Biceps, Forearms I, Total Body Workout III, Upper Body Workouts, Back, Biceps, Forearms II, Standing Exclusive, Sedentary Worker

Fun Fact: If you spend a lot of time working at a computer or typing, then the above stretches are great to use every 90 minutes or so. These limber your forearm muscle and counterbalances the positioning used while typing for hours at a time.

Hanging Upper Body
Affects: back, chest, shoulders

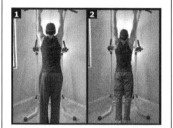

Grasp an overhead pull-up bar and lean forward. Let your upper body open up and relax while keeping your shoulder blades pinched back. When finished, carefully step forward to a standing position and release your grip.

Related programs: Back, Biceps, Forearms I, Upper Body Workouts, Back, Biceps, Forearms II, Standing Exclusive

Knee Hug
Affects: glutes, thighs, low back

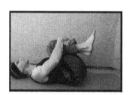

Lie on your back, bring your knees to your chest, and then hug your legs.

Related programs: Seated to Lying, Lying, Lower Body Workout, Total Hips II

Knee Hug Modification
Affects: glutes, thighs, low back

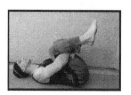

If you cannot do the knee hug, then lie on your back, and grasp under your knees.

Related programs: Seated to Lying, Lying, Lower Body Workout, Total Hips II

Kneeling Split Leg
Affects: inner thighs

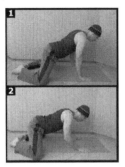

Kneel with your toes pointed outward, your knees separated away from your midline and your hands placed on the floor for support. Ease your weight into your pelvis as you push back with your hands. Slowly ease your body forward.

Related programs: Kneeling to Seated, Total Body Workout II, Kneeling Exclusive

Kneeling Hip Flexor
Affects: hip flexors, abs, side abs

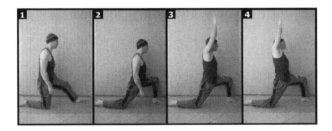

From a kneeling position, bring one leg forward, bend at the knee and place your foot flat on the floor. Place both hands on your knee and bring your posture upright. Raise the opposite arm overhead. Lean toward the side of the lead leg and slightly back. To deepen the stretch, bring your foot further forward as you leave your kneeling leg in place.

Related programs: Kneeling to Seated, Hams, Hip Flexors, Inner Thighs, Calves, Total Hips I, Total Body Workout I, Total Body Workout III, Lower Body Workout, Hams, Hip Flexors, Calves, Total Hips II, Kneeling Exclusive, Sedentary Worker

Kneeling Shoulder & Back with Chair
Affects: back, chest, shoulder

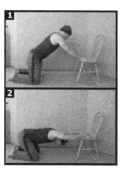

Kneel on the floor facing a chair. Place your arms on the chair and allow your upper body to hang toward the ground.

Related programs: Chest, Shoulders, Triceps, Neck, Total Body Workout I, Total Body Workout II, Chest, Shoulders, Neck, Back, Biceps, Forearms II, Kneeling Exclusive

Kneeling Thigh
Affects: quadriceps

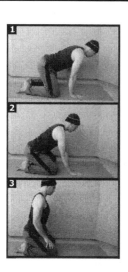

Kneel on the floor with your feet placed together behind you. Place your palms on the floor and slowly ease your butt to rest on your heels. When you can comfortably rest your butt on your heels, press your hands off the floor and bring your torso to an upright position.

Related programs: Kneeling to Seated, Total Body Workout II, Kneeling Exclusive, Sedentary Worker

Lateral Leg
Affects: inner thighs

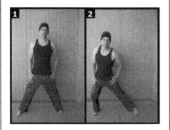

Separate your stance and keep your body upright. Bend one leg at the hip and knee while keeping the opposite leg straight. The more you lean toward your straightened leg, the deeper you feel the stretch.

Related programs: Standing Exclusive

Lying Butterfly
Affects: inner thighs

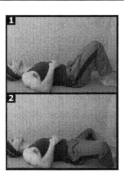

Lie on the floor, bend your knees and place your heels against each other. Allow your knees to separate and relax toward the ground. As you become more comfortable with this stretch, draw your heels closer to your inner thighs. Keep your low back flat and your arms relaxed.

Related programs: Lying

CAUTION: Anytime you complete a floor exercise and stand up, do so gradually. Roll to your side, press up to a kneeling position, pause, and then stand up.

Lying Cross Leg Twist
Affects: glutes, side abs, lower back

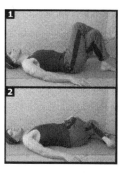

From a lying position, cross one leg over the other with your knees stacked on each other. Rest your arms outward with your palms on the ground. Turn your stacked legs away from the side of the upper leg. Look away from the direction you twist.

Related programs: Seated to Lying, Lying

Lying Figure-4
Affects: glutes

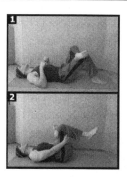

Lie on your back, cross one leg over the other with the ankle by the knee. Grasp the bottom thigh and bring to your chest.

Related programs: Lying, Total Body Workout II

Beginner's Tip: If it is impossible to cross your legs lying down, then try to do it sitting in a chair. When you sit down and cross your legs, then simply lean forward to stretch the glutes.

Lying Figure 4 Modification
Affects: glutes

Modification for excess tightness

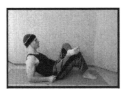

In the event of excess tightness, rather than draw the thigh into your chest, raise your upper body and support yourself on your elbows.

Related programs: Lying, Total Body Workout II

Lying Hamstring
Affects: hamstrings

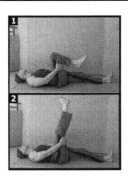

Lie on your back with your legs on the floor. Guide one knee up with your hands, and then slowly extend your leg. A soft bend in the knee is all right, however, try to keep the leg as extended and straightened as possible. If you have too much tension, then bend the opposite knee and place the foot on the floor to relieve some pressure.

Related programs: Lying

Fun Fact: The lying stretches are the best way to protect your low back. If you have a weak low back, then the lying stretches are a great starting point. Once you've mastered these stretches, move to the more difficult seated and kneeling exercises.

Neck ROM (range-of-motion)
Affects: neck

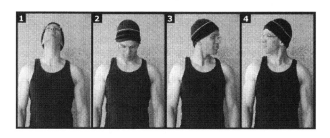

Look up and raise your chin up as high as you can and hold the position. Look down and drive the crown of your head as high as you can, and then stay. Bring your head back to neutral. Turn your chin left and hold. Then turn to the right and hold. Hold each position for 6-10 seconds.

Related programs: Chest, Shoulders, Triceps, Neck, Total Body Workout I, Total Body Workout III, Total Body Workout IV, Upper Body Workouts, Chest, Shoulders, Neck, Seated Exclusive, Standing Exclusive, Sedentary Worker

Helpful Tip: Office jobs or prolonged sitting leads to issues with the head and shoulders drifting forward, causing undue stress on the neck. Stretching the shoulders and neck should be a priority then. The Neck ROM stretch is perfect for relieving tension. Focus mostly on the upward and sideways movement and show less emphasis on the downward position.

Overhead Interlaced Palms
Affects: forearms, wrists, back, shoulders

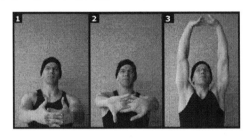

Interlace your palms, then extend your arms overhead and rotate your interlaced palms upward. Try to straighten your spine upward and lift your chin.

Related programs: Total Body Workout I, Total Body Workout II, Total Body Workout III, Total Body Workout IV, Upper Body Workouts, Chest, Shoulders, Neck, Back, Biceps, Forearms II, Chest, Triceps, Forearms, Seated Exclusive, Standing Exclusive, Sedentary Worker

Pandiculation – Active stretching commonly associated with the simultaneous stretching and yawning action upon waking[46]. Unlike the passive stretches shown throughout this book, pandiculating is an active stretch. Passive stretches feel slightly uncomfortable, whereas, active stretches can seem more pleasurable and relaxing. Experiment with the Overhead Interlaced Palms stretch and pandiculation. It can feel incredibly good and loosen up the entire body.

Overhead Triceps
Affects: triceps, back, shoulders

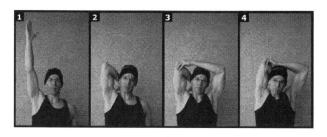

Reach one arm overhead, bend that elbow and touch the back of your neck. With your free hand, grasp your elbow overhead, guide it back and allow your hand to slide down your back. Stretch each side equally.

Related programs: Chest, Shoulders, Triceps, Neck, Total Body Workout I, Total Body Workout II, Total Body Workout IV, Seated Exclusive, Standing Exclusive

Helpful Tip: For the Overhead Triceps stretch, try to keep your shoulder blades pinched back and down throughout the exercise. Guide the elbow back and avoid pulling on the back of your arm. You could even place your elbow into the wall and lean forward for a better passive stretch.

Pigeon Pose
Affects: glutes, hip flexors, inner thigh, hamstrings

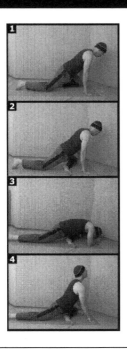

Kneel down with one knee further forward than the other. Place your extended arms directly below your shoulders for support. Bring one knee further forward as you extend the other leg behind until your knee and hip are straight, flattening your thigh into the ground. Guide your lead leg across your body on the floor until your outer ankle is resting on the ground in front of the rear-facing leg. Press upward and sink back so your inner thigh lowers to the ground.

Related programs: Kneeling to Seated, Total Hips I, Total Body Workout I, Total Body Workout III, Lower Body Workout, Total Hips II, Kneeling Exclusive, Sedentary Worker

Helpful Tip: If you are familiar with yoga, then you may recognize a few positions in this book. The pigeon is a classic yoga pose. However, it is difficult for exercise newbies. To ease into the pigeon pose, do these stretches first:

1. *Child Pose*

2. *Cobra Pose*

3. *Kneeling Hip Flexor*

4. *Lying Figure-4*

Rear Shoulder & Neck
Affects: shoulders, neck

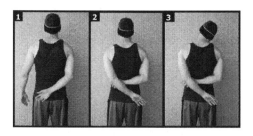

Bring one extended arm behind your back and grasp the elbow with the other hand. Pull the arm across the midline of the back. Tilt your head away from the side of the extended arm.

Related programs: Total Body Workout I, Total Body Workout III, Upper Body Workouts, Chest, Shoulders, Neck, Chest, Triceps, Forearms, Seated Exclusive, Standing Exclusive, Sedentary Worker

Fun Fact: Amazon warehouses require their employees to stretch before the shift starts and after the lunch break. They feel this minimizes the risk of injury and increases employee efficiency. Additionally, it's an excellent way to communicate pertinent information while keeping employees active before intense labor. When I worked at the Amazon warehouse, the Rear Shoulder & Neck was a staple of most stretch routines.

Reverse Hug
Affects: shoulders

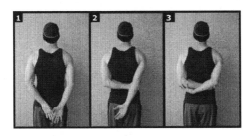

Reach both arms behind you and grasp your forearms as close to your elbows as possible. Pinch your shoulders back and down. If at first you are unable to grasp your forearms, reach behind you and clasp your hands together.

Related programs: Chest, Shoulders, Triceps, Neck, Total Body Workout I, Total Body Workout IV, Upper Body Workouts, Chest, Shoulders, Neck, Chest, Triceps, Forearms, Seated Exclusive, Standing Exclusive

Helpful Tip: If the Reverse Hug is too difficult or your shoulders are too tight to reach behind you, then the Rear Shoulder & Neck stretch is an excellent place to start. Before you do either stretch, loosen your shoulders with

1. *Wall-Assisted Chest, Shoulder & Neck*

2. *Neck ROM*

3. *Wall-Assisted Straight Arm Chest, Shoulder & Neck*

Seated Butterfly
Affects: inner thighs

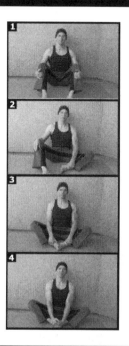

From a seated position, bend your knees and place your heels together. Grasp the top of your feet and draw your heels as close to your inner thigh as possible. Lift your big toes up as you press your knees down with your elbows. Keep your posture upright throughout the stretch and bend forward at the hips to deepen the stretch.

Related programs: Seated to Lying, Hams, Hip Flexors, Inner Thighs, Calves, Lower Body Workout, Seated Exclusive

Seated Hamstring
Affects: hamstrings

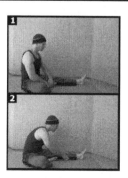

From a seated position, extend one leg out and place the other foot on your knee. Keep your posture up as your reach to the extended leg and hold the position. Stretch each side equally.

Related programs: Seated to Lying, Kneeling to Seated, Total Body Workout I, Lower Body Workout, Seated Exclusive

Seated Knee Hug
Affects: glutes, thighs, obliques

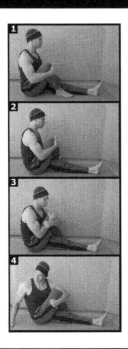

From a seated position, extend one leg and cross the other leg over with that foot placed flat on the ground. Place your heel next to the extended knee. Hug your bent knee and hold. Then, turn your torso toward the direction of the knee, put your palm on the ground and look over your shoulder.

Related programs: Seated to Lying, Total Body Workout I, Lower Body Workout, Total Hips II, Seated Exclusive

Seated Split-Leg Hamstring
Affects: hamstrings, inner thighs

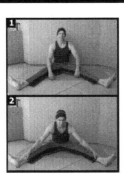

Sit on the floor with your legs extended and separated away from the midline of your body. Keep your posture up, bend forward at the hips and reach toward your feet. Grasp your legs at the furthest point and hold this position.

Related programs: Seated to Lying, Lower Body Workout, Seated Exclusive

Self Hug

Affects: shoulders, upper back

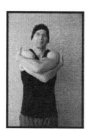

Cross your arms over your chest and hug yourself.

Related programs: Total Upper Body, Back, Biceps, Forearms I, Total Body Workout I, Total Body Workout IV, Upper Body Workouts, Chest, Shoulders, Neck, Seated Exclusive, Standing Exclusive

Side Lying Ankle Pick

Affects: quadriceps, hip flexor

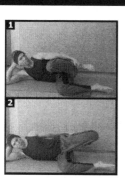

Lie on your side, bend your knee and bring forward. Grasp your ankle and pull your heel back toward your butt. Draw your leg behind you and hold. Stretch each side equally.

Related programs: Total Body Workout II, Lower Body Workout

Helpful Tip: If the Standing Ankle Pick stretch is too difficult for you to balance, then the Side Lying Ankle Pick is an adequate replacement. In both stretches, avoid grasping the top of your foot because it puts too much pressure on the knee and could cause the calf muscle to spasm.

Single Calf (pike)
Affects: calves, hamstrings

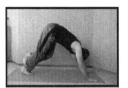

From a standing position, bend at the waist and place your palms on the ground. Keep your back straight as possible and your butt pointed upward. Lift one leg and cross the foot over the back of your weight-bearing ankle.

Related programs: Lower Body Workout, Hams, Hip Flexors, Calves

Single Knee Hug
Affects: glutes, quadriceps

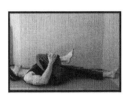

Lie on your back, bring your knee to your chest and hug it. Grasp under your knee if you are not comfortable with the single knee hug. Stretch each side equally.

Related programs: Lying

Helpful Tip: If the Lying Knee Hug is too hard, then try the Single Knee Hug as a suitable replacement. To isolate your glutes, draw your knee across your body while keeping your back flat.

Single Shoulder/Elbow Grasp

Affects: shoulders, neck

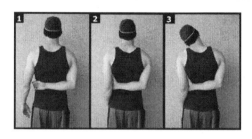

With one arm at your side, reach the other arm behind your back, and grasp the opposite elbow. Tilt your head away from the bent arm.

Related programs: Total Upper Body, Total Body Workout II, Chest, Shoulders, Neck, Chest, Triceps, Forearms, Seated Exclusive, Standing Exclusive, Sedentary Worker

Standing Ankle Pick

Affects: quadriceps

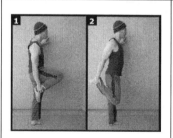

Stand near a wall and place your hand on it for support. Bend and bring your knee forward. Grasp your ankle and pull your heel to your butt. Draw your leg behind you and hold. Keep your posture upright. Stretch each side equally.

Related programs: Standing, Total Body Workout IV, Standing Exclusive

Standing Bent Hamstring
Affects: hamstrings, calves

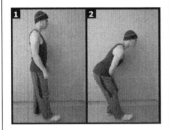

From a standing position, place one foot in front of the other. Keep the front leg straight, bend the rear leg at the waist and knee while supporting yourself above your knee. The further you drop your butt, the more you feel a stretch in the hamstrings of your extended leg. Keep your back straight throughout the stretch.

Related programs: Standing, Total Body Workout IV, Hams, Hip Flexors, Calves

Standing Cross-Legged Glute
Affects: glutes, side abs

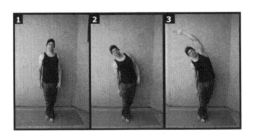

From a standing position, cross one leg in front of the other. Extend your arm upward, and then bend your torso toward the side of the lead leg. Hold this position. If the tension is too much, then keep your arms at your sides and just bend at the waist.

Related programs: Standing, Total Hips I, Total Body Workout IV, Total Hips II, Standing Exclusive, Sedentary Worker

Standing Elevated Hamstring
Affects: hamstrings, calves

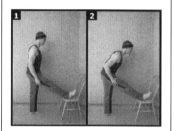

With your leg extended, place your heel onto an elevated surface in front of you. Keep your posture up, bend at the hips and grasp your leg at the furthest point.

Related programs: Hams, Hip Flexors, Calves, Standing Exclusive, Sedentary Worker

Standing Hip Flexor
Affects: hip flexors, side abs

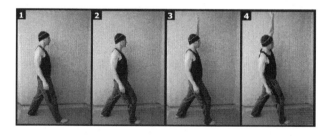

From a standing position, stagger your legs with one foot ahead of the other. Slowly bend your front knee while keeping the back knee straight. Distribute your weight equally between your legs. Visualize your belt line like a rim of a bucket and tilt the bucket backward until you feel a pull in the hip flexor of the rear leg. On the side of your rear leg, extend your arm overhead, and then lean away from that side and back.

Related programs: Standing, Total Hips I, Total Body Workout IV, Hams, Hip Flexors, Calves, Total Hips II, Standing Exclusive, Sedentary Worker

Step-Assisted Calves
Affects: calves

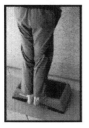	Stand with your heels hanging off a step and shift your weight slightly back.

Step-Assisted Single Calf
Affects: calves

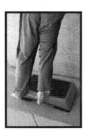	Stand with one heel hanging off a step, and the other leg extended behind you. Shift your weight slightly back, so that you feel a stretch in your calf. *Related programs: Hams, Hip Flexors, Calves, Standing Exclusive*

Bonus Stretch: A modification of the Step-Assisted Calf stretch is to use a wall. Place the balls of your feet on the wall above the baseboard. Rest your heel on the ground and gradually bend your knee toward the wall. It's okay if your toes may slip down on the wall. You will feel a great stretch in your calf muscles.

Strap Stretch: Bent Single Hamstring
Affects: hamstrings, calves

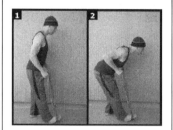

From a standing position and your feet separated, bring one foot further forward from the other. Grasp the strap ends and anchor the middle of the strap around your foot arch. Keep the front leg straight, and then bend the rear leg at the waist and knee. The further you drop your butt, the more you feel a stretch. Pull the strap back to apply additional pressure if needed.

Related programs: Hams, Hip Flexors, Inner Thighs, Calves, Strap Stretch

Strap Stretch: Chest & Shoulder
Affects: chest, shoulders

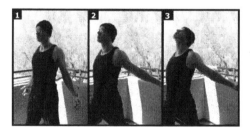

Anchor the middle of the strap to a sturdy surface, such as a pole or stationary exercise equipment. Grasp the strap ends and keep your arms at about shoulder height. Step forward and keep your arms back. Bow your chest upward and lift your chin.

Related programs: Chest, Shoulders, Triceps, Neck, Total Body Workout III, Upper Body Workouts, Chest, Shoulders, Neck, Chest, Triceps, Forearms, Sedentary Worker, Strap Stretch

Strap Stretch: Iron Cross
Affects: hamstrings, obliques, low back

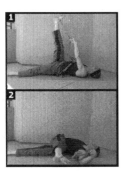

Lie on your back, place a hoop around your foot at the arch and then extend that leg upward. Grasp the strap in the opposite hand and slowly bring the leg down toward that side while keeping your upper body flat on the floor.

Related programs: Total Body Workout II, Strap Stretch

Strap Stretch: Lying Figure Four
Affects: glutes

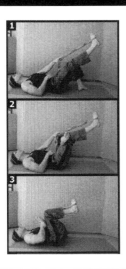

Lying on your back, place one foot on the ground with the knee bent. Cross the other leg over with the ankle next to the bent knee. Grasp the strap in both hands with the middle supported at the arch of the planted foot. Gradually pull your elbows back and upward while bringing the knee closer to your chest and keeping the resting hip flat on the floor.

Related programs: Lower Body Workout, Total Hips II, Strap Stretch

Strap Stretch: Lying Hamstring
Affects: hamstrings

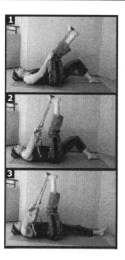

Lying on your back, grasp the strap in both hands with the middle of the strap supported on your foot arch. Bend the other knee and place that foot on the ground. Draw your knee toward your chest on the strap supported side. Extend that leg up and gently pull back on the strap to apply additional pressure. Allow the other leg to rest. For additional pressure, straighten out the leg to rest on the ground.

Related programs: Total Body Workout II, Lower Body Workout, Hams, Hip Flexors, Calves, Strap Stretch

Strap Stretch: Lying Single Thigh
Affects: quadriceps, glutes

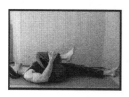

(strap not pictured)

Lying on your back, grasp the strap in both hands with the middle supported at the foot arch. Bring your bent knee to your chest. Allow the other leg to rest. Gradually pull your elbows back and upward while bringing the knee closer to your chest and keeping the resting hip flat on the floor.

Related programs: Total Hips II, Strap Stretch

Strap Stretch: Lying Split Leg Hamstring
Affects: inner thighs, hamstrings

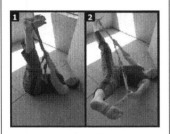

Lying on your back, place the loop ends on the arches of your feet. Extend your legs up and slowly separate them away from your midline. When finished, bend your knees toward your chest, and then place your feet flat on the floor.

Strap Stretch: Overhead Triceps
Affects: triceps, middle back, shoulders

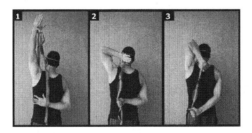

Grasp the strap with your hands about 1-2 feet apart. Bring one arm over head and bend the elbow with your hand coming to the back of your neck. Guide the other arm behind you and pull the upper arm down.

Related programs: Total Body Workout III, Upper Body Workouts, Chest, Triceps, Forearms, Strap Stretch

CAUTION: Do NOT force your arm down with the strap; merely assist.

Strap Stretch: Seated Double Hamstring
Affects: hamstrings, calves

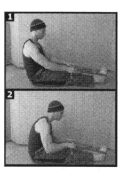

From a seated position, extend your legs together in front of you. Place the middle of the strap at your foot arches and grasp the strap ends. Keeping your posture upright, bend forward at the hip and pull your upper body toward your thighs.

Strap Stretch: Seated Single Hamstring
Affects: hamstrings, calves

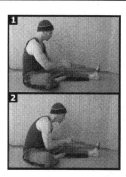

From a seated position, extend one leg in front of you and place the opposite foot into the knee of the straightened leg. Anchor the middle of the strap around the front foot arch and grasp the strap. Keeping your posture upright, lean forward and pull the strap back to apply pressure. Bring your upper body forward while keeping your back straightened.

Related programs: Hams, Hip Flexors, Inner Thighs, Calves, Strap Stretch

Helpful Tip: Keep your posture as upright as possible in all stretches.

Strap Stretch: Seated Split-Leg Hamstring
Affects: inner thighs, hamstrings

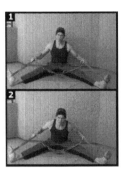

Place the loop ends of the strap over both feet at the arches. Sit on the floor with both legs extended and separated away from the midline of your body. Keep your posture upright, bend forward at the hips and reach toward your feet. Grasp the strap closest to your feet and pull your upper body forward.

Related programs: Hams, Hip Flexors, Inner Thighs, Calves, Strap Stretch

Strap Stretch: Side Lying Thigh & Hip Flexor
Affects: hip flexors, quadriceps

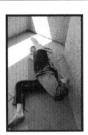

Loop one side of the strap around your foot and lie on the opposite side. Bend the bottom knee up to hip level. Bend the top leg so the heel comes toward your butt. Bring the strap behind you and over the shoulder closest to the ground. Gently pull the strap over your head or shoulder while allowing your upper hip to flex backward.

Related programs: Hams, Hip Flexors, Calves, Total Hips II, Strap Stretch

CAUTION: Avoid overarching your back when doing the Strap Stretch: Side Lying Thigh & Hip Flexor stretch. Focus on guiding the thigh behind your hip.

Wall-Assisted Butterfly
Affects: inner thighs

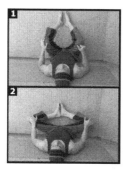

Sit with your butt against the wall, bend your knees and place your heels against each other. Allow your knees to separate toward the ground. Grasp the top of your feet and draw your heels as close to your inner thigh as possible. Lift your big toes up as you press your knees down with your elbows. Keep your posture up and proud. As you become more comfortable with this stretch, draw your heels closer to your groin.

Related programs: Total Body Workout III

Wall-Assisted Chest, Shoulder & Neck
Affects: chest, shoulders, neck

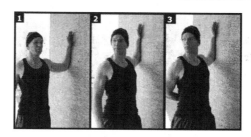

Place your elbow at shoulder height on the side closest to the wall. On the same side, step forward while planting the heel of the back leg. Pinch your shoulder blades back and turn your torso away from the wall. Turn your head away from the wall and tuck your opposite arm behind you.

Related programs: Total Upper Body, Chest, Shoulders, Triceps, Neck, Total Body Workout I, Total Body Workout II, Upper Body Workouts, Chest, Shoulders, Neck, Chest, Triceps, Forearms, Standing Exclusive, Sedentary Worker

Wall-Assisted Straight Arm Chest, Shoulder & Neck
Affects: chest, shoulders, biceps, forearms, wrists

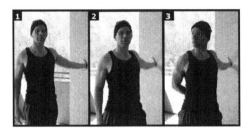

Stand within arm's reach of a wall to your side. Place your palm at shoulder height on the side closest to the wall. On the same side, step forward while keeping the heel of the back leg firmly planted. Pinch your shoulder blades back and turn your torso slightly away from the wall. Turn your head away from the wall and tuck your opposite arm behind you. Keep your posture upright at all times. Stretch each side equally.

Related programs: Back, Biceps, Forearms I, Total Body Workout IV, Upper Body Workouts, Back, Biceps, Forearms II

Wall-Assisted Single Calf
Affects: calves

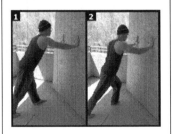

From a standing position, face two steps away from the wall. Place your palms on the wall with your arms extended. Separate your stance about shoulder-width apart and bring one foot closer to the wall with a slight bend in the knee. Extend the back leg. You will feel the stretch in the calf of the back leg. If you do not feel a stretch, separate your feet more or step further away from the wall.

Related programs: Standing, Sedentary Worker

Wall-Assisted Lying Split-Leg Hamstring
Affects: inner thighs, hamstrings

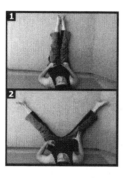

Lie on your back with your butt against the wall and your legs extended up. Separate your legs away from the midline of your body and hold the position.

Related programs: Total Body Workout III

Wall-Assisted Overhead Arm Hold
Affects: middle back, shoulders, chest

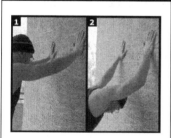

Face toward a wall within arms-reach. Extend your arms overhead and place your palms on the wall. Bend at the waist while keeping your arms above you.

Related programs: Total Upper Body, Back, Biceps, Forearms I, Total Body Workout III, Total Body Workout IV, Upper Body Workouts, Back, Biceps, Forearms II, Standing Exclusive

CAUTION: Avoid leaning too far forward in the Wall-Assisted Overhead Arm Hold. Keep your shoulder blades pinched back and bend at the hips so you bear weight on your feet and not your shoulders.

Wall-Assisted Single Leg Hamstring
Affects: hamstrings

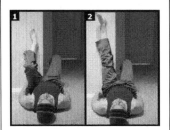

Lie down with one side of your butt close to the wall and your leg extended up. Extend the other leg on the floor. The more comfortable you become with this stretch, the closer you should move your butt toward the wall. For additional benefit, point your toes toward your knee.

Related programs: Total Body Workout III

NOTE FROM THE AUTHOR

Reading an exercise is much easier than doing it. You may stumble over some instruction or need further clarification. I encourage you to contact me should you have any questions or comments.

It means a lot to me that you invested your time and money in my content. So, I want you to get the most value possible. The last thing I wish to happen is for you to leave with questions.

The best part about sending me your questions, I can cover these concerns in future publications. And, I would even be willing to put you into my special thanks section (permitting your approval).

Send your questions to me directly at ptdale@gmail.com. I answer all of my emails and am ecstatic when I hear from you. No matter the question or concern, drop me a line.

-Dale L. Roberts

Conclusion

Stretching really is a simple yet effective method of exercise when used correctly. If you use the proper type of stretch at the right time, then you will see significant benefits that include more flexibility, mobility, safer workouts and a better overall lifestyle. You can use a brief stretch routine to maintain your joint range of motion, or you can use stretching as a standalone workout for more advantages. Either way, it's a winning situation with a little effort.

As with any exercise routine, if this is new or a change for you, then speak with your doctor about necessary modifications. Feel free to share this book and the stretch programming included to see what is best for you, and what is not appropriate to your unique health conditions.

Since I began personal training in 2006, a lot of research studies have been conducted to determine the effectiveness of stretching and what is best for your health. In due time, more scientific evidence will surface on the benefits of stretching. For now, all we have are theories and individual testimonies. Ultimately, it's up to you on what you find to be best for your health. If you wish to err on the side of caution, then I would advise you, at least, to entertain exercise methods that encourage functional flexibility in Yoga, Tai Chi, and Qigong.

The most important lesson is to try stretching, see what works for you, and build on it. With diligent and consistent practice, you may improve your health and feel all the better for it. If you are relatively new to stretching, then add these exercises a little at a time. When you comfortably perform ten to fifteen minutes at a time, you are fast on track to getting improved flexibility. You can then scale up your efforts to include the standalone routines. And, that's when simple stretching can have a significant impact on your health and fitness. Good luck to you and happy stretching!

Thank You

Thank you for taking the time to read my book. I hope that you enjoyed reading it as much as I enjoyed writing it. I have only one request; if you did like it, please leave a review. Reviews are the lifeblood of indie and small press authors and greatly help us get more books in front of more readers. If you didn't like it, that's fine too. Just leave an honest review, that's all I ask. Drop me a review on Amazon.com.

As you work toward your goals, you may have questions or run into some issues. I'd like to be able to help you, so let's connect. I don't charge for the assistance, so feel free to connect with me on the internet at:

DaleLRoberts.com

Like me on Facebook:

http://www.facebook.com/authordaleroberts

Follow me on Instagram:

http://www.instagram.com/dalelroberts

Follow me on Twitter:

http://www.twitter.com/ptdaleroberts

Subscribe to my YouTube channel:

http://www.youtube.com/ptdalelroberts

Thank you, again! I hope to hear from you and wish you the best.

-Dale

P.S. You will find my entire catalog of books on Amazon Author Central at amazon.com/author/daleroberts. Click the "Follow" button to get updates any time I publish a new book.

About The Author

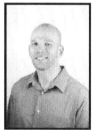

My name is Dale Lewis Roberts and I'm an American Council on Exercise Personal Trainer, Certified, with an ACE Specialty Certification in Senior Fitness. Since beginning my personal training career in 2006, I have earned numerous certifications in personal training, yoga, nutritional coaching, among others. I have worked with hundreds of clients with a variety of health & fitness goals.

While my greatest passions are health & fitness, writing and reading, I also love to spend time traveling with my wife, watching pro wrestling and playing guitar. I currently reside in Phoenix, Arizona, with my wife, Kelli, and our rescue cat, Izzie.

Subscribe to my blog at DaleLRoberts.com for all the latest posts on health and fitness tips. This is also one of the best ways to connect with me directly. Please, remember that whatever you do in life, make sure that you do what you love. Stay happy, healthy and strong!

Take a look at my catalog of books at DaleLRoberts.com/My-Book-Shelf.

Special Thanks

To my wife, Kelli - Your undying support and love give me unbelievable strength and confidence.

To my editor, Colleen Schlea - Your patience, time and dedication bring my writing to an all new level. I have seen what my books look like without you and it isn't pretty. "Thanks" doesn't even begin to express my extreme gratitude for your guidance and hand in my early-life development.

And to my number one fan and great friend, Carol Langkamp - You asked for it, now you finally get it. This is my most comprehensive coverage of stretching so that you limber up to move more freely and dance your heart out.

Kevin Allen – man, you came from out of nowhere and have been my biggest supporter and accountability partner.

Jason Bracht – no words describe my gratitude for all your coaching and guidance. I wouldn't be where I'm at if it weren't for you. Thank you, man.

Extra big thanks to Philip & Natalia Carnevale for your consultation. This project wouldn't have been as strong without you. Please take a little extra time check out Philip Carnevale photography at http://www.philipcarnevalephotography.com/.

And, Geo & Robbie for assisting behind the scenes; I appreciate your work much more than you know. Additionally, take a look at Georgej Designs, the best in fashion design, at http://www.georgejdesigns.com/.

ATTENTION: Get Your Free Gift

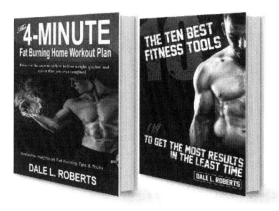

Are you interested in learning how to incinerate a ton of fat in very little time? You are not alone! Millions of people all over the world are trying to lose weight and do so in a safe and effective manner.

What I have done is put together two FREE reports to get you started on the road to success. These reports won't be up forever, so get them before they are taken down. It's my simple way of saying thank you for buying this book. To get these great reports, go to:

http://DaleLRoberts.com/4minutes

Download the reports on "The 4-Minute Fat Burning Home Workout Plan" and "The Ten Best Fitness Tools (To Get You More Results in the Least Time)" ABSOLUTELY FREE. The tips in these reports will help you lose weight, melt off fat, and get in great shape!

References

[1] Schwartz, Linda. (2015). The Dangers of Stretching. Retrieved from http://healthyliving.azcentral.com/dangers-stretching-18771.html

[2] Quill, Scott. (2015). The Truth Behind 7 Muscle Myths: Stretching Prevents Injuries. Retrieved from http://www.menshealth.com/mhlists/muscle_myths_debunked/Stretchin g_Prevents_Injuries.php

[3] Dreyfuss, Ira. (2015, March 28). Center for Disease Control: Stretching Causes Muscle Injuries. Retrieved from http://www.drmikemarshall.com/CenterforDiseaseControl_StretchingCau sesMuscleInjuries.html

[4] Inverarity, Laura. (2014, December 16). Stretching 101. Retrieved from http://physicaltherapy.about.com/od/flexibilityexercises/a/stretchbasics.h tm

[5] McGraw-Hill Concise Dictionary of Modern Medicine. (2015, April 12). Definition of flexibility. Retrieved from http://medical-dictionary.thefreedictionary.com/flexibility

[6] MedicineNet, Inc. (2012, March 19). Definition of Range of Motion. Retrieved from http://www.medicinenet.com/script/main/art.asp?articlekey=5208

[7] U.S. National Library of Medicine. (2015, June 15). Aging changes in the bones - muscles - joints. Retrieved from http://www.nlm.nih.gov/medlineplus/ency/article/004015.htm

[8] Bell, R.D., & Hoshizaki, T.B. (1981, December 6). Relationships of age and sex with range of motion of seventeen joint actions in humans. Canadian Journal of Applied Sport Sciences, pg. 202–206.

[9] Doriot, N., & Wang, X. (2006, February 22). Effects of age and gender on maximum voluntary range of motion of the upper body joints. Ergonomics, pg. 269–281.

[10] Kravitz, Len. (2009, October 26). Stretching-A Research Retrospective. Retrieved from

http://www.ideafit.com/fitness-library/stretching-research-retrospective

[11] National Center for Biotechnology Information. (1993, October 25). The physical condition of elderly women differing in habitual physical activity. Retrieved from http://www.ncbi.nlm.nih.gov/pubmed/8231760

[12] Ingraham, Paul. (2015, April 23). The Trouble with Chairs. Retrieved from https://www.painscience.com/articles/chair-trouble.php

[13] Mayo Foundation for Medical Education and Research. (2014, March 4). Stretching: Focus on flexibility. Retrieved from http://www.mayoclinic.org/healthy-lifestyle/fitness/in-depth/stretching/art-20047931

[14] Miller-Keane Encyclopedia and Dictionary of Medicine, Nursing, and Allied Health, Seventh Edition. (2003). Definition of mobility. Retrieved from http://medical-dictionary.thefreedictionary.com/mobility

[15] Murray, Jessica. (2013, May 16). Issues Impacting Work-Life Quality for People with

Mobility Limitations Living in New York City (Part 2). Retrieved from http://opencuny.org/jmurray/files/2014/03/Issues-Impacting-WLQ-for-People-with-Mobility-Limitations-in-NYC.pdf

[16] Disabella, Vincent N. (2013, June 14). Elbow and Forearm Overuse Injuries. Retrieved from http://emedicine.medscape.com/article/96638-overview

[17] Segen's Medical Dictionary. (2015, April 13). Definition of stretching. Retrieved from http://medical-dictionary.thefreedictionary.com/stretching

[18] Walsh, Kelle. (2008, June). STRETCH AND REACH: THE UNEXAGGERATED TRUTH ABOUT STRETCHING. Retrieved from https://experiencelife.com/article/stretch-and-reach-the-unexaggerated-truth-about-stretching/

[19] StretchMate, Inc. (n.d.). Flexibility & Stretching. Retrieved from http://www.stretchmate.net/stretching.htm on 2015, July 2.

[20] Spriggs, Brenda B. (2014, December 17). What causes muscle stiffness? 15 possible conditions. Retrieved from

http://www.healthline.com/symptom/muscle-stiffness

21 Mayo Foundation for Medical Education and Research. (2014, March 4). Stretching: Focus on flexibility. Retrieved from http://www.mayoclinic.org/healthy-lifestyle/fitness/in-depth/stretching/art-20047931

22 Cheffy, Sarah. (2004, February 19). ACE Lists Top Ten Reasons to Stretch. Retrieved from https://www.acefitness.org/about-ace/press-room/325/ace-lists-top-ten-reasons-to-stretch/

23 Cespedes, Andrea. (2014, February 2). Does Stretching Burn Calories? Retrieved from http://www.livestrong.com/article/438404-does-stretching-burn-calories/

24 Inverarity, Laura. (2014, December 14). Stretching 101. Retrieved from http://physicaltherapy.about.com/od/flexibilityexercises/a/stretchbasics.htm

25 Matthews, Michael. (n.d.). The Science of Stretching: Stretching and Strength, Speed, And Muscle Growth. Retrieved from http://www.muscleforlife.com/stretching-before-aerobic-exercise-or-weightlifting-yes-or-no/

26 Medical Dictionary for the Health Professions and Nursing. (2012). Definition of static exercise. Retrieved from http://medical-dictionary.thefreedictionary.com/static+exercise

27 Thacker, SB, et al. (2004, March). The impact of stretching on sports injury risk: a systematic review of the literature. Retrieved from http://www.ncbi.nlm.nih.gov/pubmed/15076777

28 McCully, Kevin. (2009, October 24). The Influence of Passive Stretch on Muscle Oxygen Saturation. Retrieved from http://link.springer.com/chapter/10.1007/978-1-4419-1241-1_45

29 Blahnik, Jay. (2011). Full-Body Flexibility, Second Edition. Retrieved from http://www.humankinetics.com/excerpts/excerpts/types-of-stretches

30 Walsh, Kelle. (2008, June). Stretch and Reach: The Unexaggerated

Truth About Stretching. Retrieved from
https://experiencelife.com/article/stretch-and-reach-the-unexaggerated-tr
uth-about-stretching/

[31] Braun, W., Sforzo, G. (2011). Delayed Onset Muscle Soreness (DOMS).
Retrieved from
https://www.acsm.org/docs/brochures/delayed-onset-muscle-soreness-(d
oms).pdf

[32] Lund, H., Vestergaard-Poulsen, P., Kanstrup, IL, Sejrsen, P. (1998,
August 8). The effect of passive stretching on delayed onset muscle
soreness, and other detrimental Affects following eccentric exercise.
Retrieved from http://www.ncbi.nlm.nih.gov/pubmed/9764443

[33] Schrier, I. (1999, October 9). Stretching before exercise does not reduce
the risk of local muscle injury: a critical review of the clinical and basic
science literature. Retrieved from
http://www.ncbi.nlm.nih.gov/pubmed/10593217

[34] Gergley, JC. (2013, April 27). Acute effect of passive static stretching on
lower-body strength in moderately trained men. Retrieved from
http://www.ncbi.nlm.nih.gov/pubmed/22692125

[35] Simic, L., et al. (2013, March 23). Does pre-exercise static stretching
inhibit maximal muscular performance? A meta-analytical review.
Retrieved from http://www.ncbi.nlm.nih.gov/pubmed/22316148

[36] Walsh, Kelle. (2008, June). Stretch and Reach: The Unexaggerated
Truth About Stretching. Retrieved from
https://experiencelife.com/article/stretch-and-reach-the-unexaggerated-tr
uth-about-stretching/

[37] Witvrouw, E., et al. (2007, April). The role of stretching in tendon
injuries. Retrieved from
http://www.ncbi.nlm.nih.gov/pmc/articles/PMC2658965/

[38] McGrath, Christopher. (2013, October 3). Family Health: Why You
Should Be Foam Rolling. Retrieved from
https://www.acefitness.org/acefit/healthy-living-article/59/3543/why-you
-should-be-foam-rolling/

[39] McDonagh, Melissa. (n.d.). Foam Rollers and Myofascial Adhesions.

Retrieved from
http://www.mccc.edu/~behrensb/documents/foamrollersMMcD2.pdf

[40] About.com. (2015, April 23). How to Use a Foam Roller for Myofascial
Release. Retrieved from
http://sportsmedicine.about.com/od/flexibilityandstretching/ss/FoamRol
ler.htm

[41] Healey, K., Et al. (2011, March). The Affects of Foam Rolling on
Myofasical Release and Performance. Retrieved from
http://journals.lww.com/nsca-jscr/Abstract/2011/03001/The_Affects_of
_Foam_Rolling_on_Myofascial_Release.45.aspx

[42] MacDonald, G.Z., Et al. (2013, March). An Acute Bout of Self-Myofascial
Release Increases Range of Motion Without a Subsequent Decrease in
Muscle Activation or Force. Retrieved from
http://journals.lww.com/nsca-jscr/Abstract/2013/03000/An_Acute_Bout
_of_Self_Myofascial_Release_Increases.34.aspx

[43] Okamoto, T., Et al. (2014, January). Acute Affects of Self-Myofascial
Release Using a Foam Roller on Arterial Function. Retrieved from
http://journals.lww.com/nsca-jscr/Abstract/2014/01000/Acute_Affects_
of_Self_Myofascial_Release_Using_a.9.aspx

[44] Southern Connecticut Muscle & Joint Performance Chiropractic. (n.d.).
Staying Healthy with Foam Rolling. Retrieved from
http://www.branfordchiropractor.com/2014/09/24/staying-healthy-with-
foam-rolling/ on 2015, July 2.

[45] Gale Encyclopedia of Medicine. (2015, April 24). Definition of
hypermobility. Retrieved from
http://medical-dictionary.thefreedictionary.com/hypermobility

[46] Conjecture Corporation. (n.d.). What is Pandiculation? Retrieved on
2016, January 30 from
http://www.wisegeek.com/what-is-pandiculation.htm

Made in the USA
San Bernardino, CA
02 July 2017